STRESS LESS

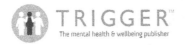

ENDORSEMENTS

"Teenagers are really stressed these days – and finally someone who actually IS a teen has written a fantastic book that's grounded in science while also being super practical and helpful. Every teenager will get a lot out of this book (and their parents, too)."

> – Rick Hanson, Ph.D., psychologist and *New York Times* best-selling author of *Hardwiring Happiness*

"I met Adam Avin many years ago and experienced him as an old soul with a wise mind and loving heart. He was the first teen to attend and complete my 10-Week Certificate Professional Training Program. Since then, he has been an inspiration to me – watching him see a need to help children and teens at such a young age has been awe-inspiring. The knowledge he imparts in *Stress Less* is nothing short of amazing. He weaves throughout this book a patchwork of ways to help a teen grow, learn and change. I wholeheartedly and without one ounce of reservation recommend this book to teens, parents and helping professionals to learn from someone who is not only an expert, but a teen."

> – Gina Biegel, MA, LMFT, creator of the Mindfulness-Based Stress Reduction for Teens (MBSR-T) and Stressed Teens programs

"Adam Avin is a powerful advocate for mindfulness, mental health and his generation. In these pages you'll find many different tools to overcome stress and other challenges, from a fellow young perspective sharing directly from his own lived experience."

– Dr. Christopher Willard, clinical psychologist, author and lecturer at Harvard Medical School

STRESS LESS:
Mindfulness for Teenagers

ADAM AVIN

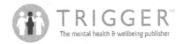

TRIGGER™
The mental health & wellbeing publisher

Published in 2023 by Trigger Publishing
An imprint of Shaw Callaghan Ltd
UK Office
The Stanley Building
7 Pancras Square
Kings Cross
London N1C 4AG

US Office
On Point Executive Center, Inc
3030 N. Rocky Point Drive W.
Suite 150
Tampa, FL 33607
www.triggerhub.org

A CIP catalogue record for this book is available upon request
from the British Library
ISBN: 978-1-83796-999-9
Ebook ISBN: 978-1-83796-241-9

To anyone reading this book,
please know you're not alone.

TABLE OF CONTENTS

FOREWORD
BY UDONIS HASLEM

Wow, what I would have given to have a book like this when I was growing up. From mindfulness techniques to journaling breaks to self-compassion practices, Adam has provided so many helpful activities to keep you in the driver's seat when dealing with stress and difficult emotions. I have been using some of these tips and tricks before I knew they had official names, so let's just say this book hits home for me.

Growing up in Liberty City, Florida, wasn't the easiest. If you took the bus at night and didn't run home from your stop, you could instead run into trouble – getting beaten up, robbed or worse. I also didn't grow up with my mom, which was really hard, but she was battling her own demons, namely addiction. Through pure determination, she eventually got clean, and in my adulthood, we began to form a relationship. Sadly, just as we started to reconnect, cancer struck, and she passed away in 2012. With everything she went through, hands down, she was the strongest person I have ever known. But between my environment and not having my mother around, I wasn't the easiest to raise.

I was an "all-hands-on-deck" kind of kid. I always seemed to have the right intentions, but I made mistakes and got into trouble. I was raised by my dad and stepmother, Barbara, but my dad also struggled with addiction, so Barbara was the one that really stepped up as the steady and reliable parent throughout my childhood. She gave me everything I needed and more. The thing is, though, even with someone as wonderful as Barbara in my life, because addiction, crime and homelessness surrounded me, I thought that was the norm.

It wasn't until I enrolled at Miami Senior High School that I began to take basketball seriously. I realized that I could use it to break the cycle and create a different life for myself. Before then, I lived one day at a time. Maybe it was because, in my world, one mistake could cost you your freedom, or even your life. I witnessed it every day. I didn't realize until I started college that everyone didn't grow up like me. Reflecting on my journey, I know that I must be here for a reason – a reason much bigger than basketball.

I credit my late stepbrother, Sam, for introducing me to basketball. He was the one who used to take me to the courts to play against the older guys. When we lost him in 1999 to HIV/AIDS, I was a mess. Not only did I lose someone I loved and admired, but I had to lie about how and why he died. You see, at that time, HIV/AIDS was still very stigmatized. It was a source of discrimination, riddled with misconceptions. I am proud of how far both treatment and understanding of HIV/AIDS have come. Today, with the proper care and medication, people with HIV can live long and healthy lives and never develop AIDS.

While it was incredibly hard to know the truth and not be able to speak about it, I was determined to not let the sadness or anger take over. I talked to trusted family, friends and coaches to get my emotions out and, of course, I had basketball, which helped. I now focus on the gratitude – I am forever grateful for the time I had with Sam, and the patience he had with me while I shot airballs he confidently called passes.

The road to success is not easy, and I had plenty of bumps along the way. There will be many points where you fall and have to get back up to try again. Those are the moments that define success, that separate the winners from the rest. Because high school and college basketball showered me with praise, one of those defining moments for me was the 2002 NBA Draft.

Just before the draft, an NBA head coach told me that if I was still available at the time of their second-round pick, they would draft me. I was excited; I had worked so hard for so long, and it was finally all going to pay off. My friends and family were just as excited. We planned to watch the draft at home together and then go out and celebrate. Everything was set up for a night I would never forget. And for better or worse, that was true. I will never forget that night – but not for the reasons I had thought.

I didn't get drafted, and it was the first time that basketball didn't take me where I wanted to go.

I thought I had done everything right. I had an impressive basketball resume, practiced the hardest year-round and kept myself out of trouble throughout college, more or less. I also had all the hype – I was named All-SEC First Team twice, I held college records, and we made it to the NCAA Tournament all four years I played at Florida. I thought I had done everything I was supposed to do as a player, and that my highlights, awards and character spoke for themselves.

I started playing in a Pro Summer League after going undrafted, thinking – knowing – I was better than almost all the draft picks playing alongside me. The NBA just didn't agree. I was chronically upset and disappointed that entire summer, and that opened my eyes – and helped me change course. Instead of complaining, whining and blaming coaches or the NBA, I took a step back and reevaluated everything that I could control, influence and change.

Once I was able to process my emotions, I was able to make decisions that weren't reaction-based. I have always been the type of person who believes that when one door closes, another door opens, and I truly believed that a kid from Liberty City could fulfill his dreams. I knew I could play and didn't want to give up just because I didn't get drafted.

About a month later, I accepted a position with the Élan Chalon basketball team in Chalon-sur-Saône, France. I was determined to use that opportunity to prepare for another shot at the NBA. Don't get me wrong, I gave myself one night to have a pity party, but at the end of the day, I had to ask myself, "What can I do differently this time? What do I need to do to get the NBA to see what I know to be true about myself?" I treated my time in France like a business trip, and I even stayed on Eastern time throughout the season. I never got comfortable because I knew if I did, I could get complacent.

You may be reading this thinking, "So, you didn't get drafted, but look at you now. Twenty seasons in the NBA, with the *same* team, *and* helping your hometown community." You have to remember, though, at that time, in 2002, I had no idea what my future held. I was lost and confused. I needed to get through that dark place I had found myself in.

I knew I had the heart, grind and ability to make it and I always gave it my all. For me, the play isn't over until you hear the whistle – that's how I've always operated. I simply needed to trust myself and focus on my goal. Because physical health is directly correlated to mental health, I dialed up my conditioning workouts and improved my food choices. I took full advantage of everything I had while in France and put myself in the best position I could to make the jump to the NBA.

When I finally signed with the Miami HEAT in 2003, I still felt like I had so much to prove as a both a basketball player and person. I just wanted to keep my head down and do the work. What I didn't realize initially was that being able to play alongside some of the greatest in the game and learn from their experiences was priceless. D-Wade showed me how to get out of my comfort zone, LeBron sharpened my basketball IQ, CB taught me about patience, and Shaq stressed the importance of sticking to a routine and believing in myself no matter what anyone else said. Erik Spoelstra and Pat Riley instilled more in me over one season than I ever imagined possible.

Pat once said, "Hard work doesn't guarantee anything, but without it you don't have a chance." And I repeat this quote all the time, especially when I speak to teens. If you want to reach your potential, you really have to work hard to get there. I went from being a rookie with a chip on my shoulder in 2003, to winning a Chip with my teammates in 2006.

I am telling you this because I truly believe each of you deserves the opportunity to be successful and thrive in all aspects of your lives; however, navigating your way can be overwhelming and daunting. The reason I care so much about helping others, including you, is because I was fortunate enough to have family, friends and coaches who were there for me when I needed them the most. Sometimes, you will need somebody to point you in the right direction or to give you advice you didn't know you needed. When that time comes, take the help; it's okay to get a boost from someone who cares.

There is absolutely no downside in asking for help, and no reason to be embarrassed. As adults, it's our responsibility to help teens like you grow up strong and confident. It doesn't even need to be a close friend or family member; a casual conversation with someone in a place to help, or just listen, can make a great difference.

I know that there is no quick fix for anxiety, depression or overall mental clarity and "happiness." Life is not a predictable path and honestly, that would be boring. It is a journey that can be exciting and scary at the same time. Personally, I have found mindfulness as a helpful tool, using it to create daily rituals and positive habits. I consciously set aside time to play with my dogs, and in the mornings, I list reasons to be grateful and more present and aware. (Hint: Writing it down makes it easier to do daily.) I've had a friend tell me they do mirror affirmations while holding their dog and talking positively about themselves – to themselves – in the mirror. It sounds silly, but if you repeat phrases like, "I am smart," "I am worthy," "I am a great friend," and "I am doing my best," over and over again, you will start to believe what you're saying.

I find that when I do these small rituals consistently, I stay more balanced and present, and less anxious. Next time you're feeling down, whether you know why or not, try one of these suggestions, and I bet you'll end up with a smile on your face. By taking control of your story and practicing positive self-talk, you will be able to improve your internal conversations over time. The key, though, is to practice these rituals even when the times are good. This helps you hold on to gratitude for what you have and prepare for the tough times that may come. When I look back at my career and how far I've come, it's clear my internal and external habits paved the way for my success.

Adversity and challenges are part of everyone's life. Unfortunately, I know a lot of young people are ashamed to speak about mental health. But let's end the stigma. Take care of your mind. Work on your inner thoughts and be kind to yourself and your brain. Look for the people who are willing to help. Enjoy and use this book, practice the mindfulness exercises, and then practice them again and again – mindfulness, just like basketball, requires practice. You practice getting ready for a game the same as you practice mindfulness to strengthen your thoughts. After you've read this book, spread the word, share it with a friend. Let this be the beginning of your journey to a fulfilling future.

Now, I give my time and energy to others both on a personal level and through the Udonis Haslem Foundation because it's all about paying it forward. Regardless of circumstance, every person needs grace and compassion. I know it may not always be easy, but starting your journey is truly the hardest part. Life can be better than what you may wake up to and see, so think of every day as a new opportunity. I have never forgotten where I came from and have worked every day to turn my experiences into opportunities to help others. Honestly, I attribute a good amount of my grit, morals and mental toughness to growing up in Liberty City.

Adam has been an advocate for mental health since he was nine, but what impresses me the most isn't that he's given a TEDx Talk or founded a non-profit before his teenage years; it's his character, because you can't teach character. He's a selfless individual who wants to make this world a better place and he gives without expecting anything in return. People like Adam are the real MVPs. Fortunately for me, we crossed paths, and I am able to combine two core pillars of my foundation (helping children and advocating for mental health) with his platform. I am forever thankful to have been given the opportunity to work with Adam and continue to help others navigate their own mental health challenges.

Thank you, Adam. Thank you for allowing me to be a part of this chapter in your life. I am excited for this new friendship and for what the future holds for you and every teen that is doing their part to make our world a better place.

And remember, don't let setbacks define you. Use them as learning experiences to help you grow and become stronger.

Keep your head up,
UD

INTRODUCTION

Okay, so, you're probably wondering, *"Why should I spend my time reading this book?"*

I get it, believe me.

I'd rather spend my time hanging out with friends, playing video games, watching sports, listening to music and – my favorite – eating cookies. Like so many teens, I feel stressed and overwhelmed by having to get good grades and get into college; lonely when I'm bored and have no one to talk to; and frustrated when my parents tell me what to do or ask me so many questions that I feel like I'm on trial.

We can all probably agree that teens aren't known for being able to pause and respond (instead of reacting to things). Most of us are more prone to fire sarcastic comments or roll our eyes if we get annoyed. I don't know about you, but although I consider myself a mindful teen, I've definitely been at the point where I've wanted to scream sometimes. I know that we usually "don't want to hear it," and that maybe we think we have the answers, but we don't. My Grandpa Alan used to say that we are never too old to learn and that he learned something new every single day, up until the day he died at 74. Sometimes, I have to remind myself of that when I'm having one of those moments. But I also think that adults and professionals who work with teens should understand that we have an intrinsic inner strength and resilience; we simply need to be taught how to recognize and appreciate the power inside to develop an "I've got this – everything is okay" mindset.

As I write this, I'm still in high school, and I'm also a mental health education advocate, which means that I teach others about mindfulness and do a lot of public speaking. Even though

I love this role, I used to get nervous when I had to speak in front of large crowds. Luckily, over the years, I've learned how to cope when I feel this and other types of stress: by practicing techniques that help me let go of negative feelings and live a calmer, more mindful life. I want to share my methods with you because they're all great ways to deal with the stress and emotions we feel as teens, often stemming from:

- Hormones
- School stress
- Peer pressure
- Social media
- Bullying
- A lack of self-confidence
- Isolation.

The tools I share in this book can help you feel a sense of calm and control in these areas and more. And, once you learn these techniques, you can continue to rely on them to deal with stress as you get older, too.

ABOUT THE BOOK

I want teens to know that they're not alone in the world. There are many strategies that can transform stress, anxiety, sadness or anger into kindness, self-love, confidence and compassion. My friend, Laura Bakosh, co-founder of the mindfulness program Inner Explorer, says that we have to train our brains, just like we do when we go to the gym to train our bodies. On top of that, she says we should take care of our mental health just like we take care of our oral health by brushing our teeth every day.

Unfortunately, none of the things you'll learn in this book are going to magically fix your life so that you're happy 100 percent of the time. However, I guarantee if you find some techniques that resonate with you and you practice them – even for five minutes a day – they can be magic, and when you truly need them, you'll have the right tools.

These tools incorporate both mindfulness and social-emotional learning, which I think are the secrets to a happier and healthier life. **Mindfulness** means that we focus on what's happening right now, rather than thinking about the past or worrying about the future. **Social-emotional learning (SEL)** means that we become aware of ourselves and others so we can regulate our emotions. Putting them together, we've got **mindfulness-based social-emotional learning (MBSEL)**. These skills train our brains to make choices that will, in turn, make us more aware, accepting, compassionate and kind, both to ourselves and others.

To work toward that goal, I have shared several mindful activities and practices in boxes throughout this book for you to try. I've also included self-reflection prompts for journaling breaks, a practice that will help you explore your emotions, actions and reactions, so be sure to have a journal or notebook handy as you read. Finally, I've highlighted more activities in grey outside of the boxes for you to try if you'd like.

My hope is that this book can help you deal with stress and emotions in a way that works for you, while creating a space for some happiness and inner peace amid all the crazy in the world. If what you read helps you get through the next argument with a friend without saying something you'll later regret, finish a family dinner without grinding your teeth, or evade a screaming match with a younger sibling, then I've done my job.

ABOUT ME

My Great-Grandpa Jack taught me that the mind controls the body (and vice versa), and our mindset can help us to be happier and healthier and have a more balanced life. When he passed away, I wanted to honor him by teaching others about his mindful mindset.

With the help of my mom Marni, when I was about nine years old, I started a non-profit organization called the Wuf Shanti Children's Wellness Foundation, through which I teach mindfulness and social-emotional learning to young kids and teens. Then, when I was 14, I founded the Kids' Association for Mindfulness in Education and the Mindful Kids Peace Summit. I am certified in Mindfulness-Based Stress Reduction for Teens, Kidding Around Yoga, and the Emotion Code, and was the youngest meditation instructor at Yoga International and Inner Explorer. I also had the honor to present a TEDx Youth Talk about getting mindful and social-emotional learning programs into our education system, during which I spoke about why mental health education is key to stopping violence, and how we can use our voices to make a positive difference in the world.

ABOUT WUF SHANTI

When I first started Wuf Shanti, we focused a lot on yoga, breathing and meditations, but as I grew up, so did Wuf Shanti. My vocabulary evolved, and our curriculum expanded from classes for 3-to-10-year-olds led by a dog character, to a more serious program shared with 11-to-17-year-olds in middle and high schools. The topics we cover – many of which I'll touch on in this book – include:

- Diversity and inclusion
- Communication
- Kindness and empathy

- Anti-bullying
- Stress reduction
- Positive psychology
- Connection and collaboration
- Self-compassion
- Substance abuse
- Suicide prevention
- Mental health.

Wuf Shanti's teachings center on both the self – that we are all special and worthy of love as our authentic selves – and our connections to others, which we can forge with kindness, compassion and empathy.

Wuf Shanti's mission is to teach the next generation how to have a mindful mindset, express gratitude and spread kindness, by encouraging kids and teens to live in health and wellness, peace and positivity, and teaching them the tools to deal with stress in order to make this world a better place. Our intent is to get MBSEL programs into classrooms for kids of all ages, so that all of them – from kindergartners to high school seniors – learn to cope with emotions and reduce self-harm and violence to others. My goal is for kids and teens to grow up less depressed and anxious, and more compassionate and empathetic.

HOW I GOT STARTED

I'm lucky to have had awesome role models in my life. They listened and shared their wisdom since I was very young. As I mentioned, my journey started with my Great-Grandpa Jack. He didn't actively practice yoga or meditation, but he lived mindfully, and he taught me mindfulness at an early age. I remember when I was about three, Grandpa Jack was holding my hand as we walked on the Miami Beach Boardwalk. He said, "Breathe in the ocean air. What do you smell? Listen to the birds. What are they saying?" As we walked, he would smile at everyone that passed, and then he would turn to me and say, "Smile, and the world will smile with you." Beyond that, Grandpa Jack would always repeat to me, "Think well to be well." He truly believed that our minds control our bodies, and that we can choose to be happier. He'd look at himself in the mirror, pat his cheeks and smile, and say, "I love myself." If I got frustrated with something, he'd smile and say, "Breathe and patience." This is how I grew up learning the skills I now teach.

My Grandpa Alan (Great-Grandpa Jack's son) and I were very close as well. He was one of the smartest and kindest men I've ever known, and he was constantly teaching me valuable lessons, too. One time, when he was nearing the end of his battle with cancer, he sat me down and took out his phone, which had his notes on it, and he started reading off some driving tips that he'd written down. I asked why he was talking to me about that since I wasn't turning 16 for another month, and he said that he may not be here by then, so he wanted to make sure that we had talked about something that would be such a big deal in my life before he was gone.

Grandpa Alan always believed that we shouldn't sweat the small stuff… and everything was small stuff. I asked him how he could be so positive in the midst of his cancer diagnosis. He said, "Well, to be honest, I've tried getting to positive. I have always been known for my optimism and positive attitude, but that doesn't mean being blind to realities. So, I decided to get to neutral."

This was a poignant lesson for me. There is something between negative and positive. It's neutral. And to me, that's balance. We don't have to be happy all the time. We can feel our feelings, and then we can learn to cope with them. I understood that Grandpa couldn't be happy about what was going on in his life, but he got to a place of acceptance for what he couldn't change, and gratitude for the life he'd had and the time we were spending together at that moment.

Gratitude was a tenet of my Great-Grandpa Jack's teachings, too. He'd often say, "Smile and say thank you." An attitude of gratitude can change the vibration of the world. Writing this makes me remember that, when I was younger, every night before bedtime, my mom would ask, "What are you grateful for today?" She did this to show me that, no matter what tragedy I thought had occurred that day, I could always find something good to counteract it, even if it was just that the sun was shining or the dog had greeted me with a very happily wagging tail.

So, back to this book:

Admittedly, I don't love when people lecture to me, so I'm going to do my best throughout this book to make sure that this doesn't sound like a lecture.

My Grandma Nola likes to remind us of the Golden Rule: "Do unto others as you'd have done unto you." In other words, it tells us to treat others the way that we want to be treated because it helps us to make and keep friends.

This is a good rule, but not just for how we treat others – it's also the way we should treat ourselves.

You would never allow your phone battery to get down to zero percent without making sure it's charged, so don't allow your body and mind to get down to zero percent either. And on my end, I promise not to tell you to "just breathe," and I won't suggest that you always have to be happy. After all, mindfulness doesn't mean ignoring how you feel – instead, it's the key to self-awareness, self-acceptance, healthy coping and navigating stress.

I believe that we get to feel what we feel, and we can choose how we handle it and express it. "Think well to be well" no longer means "think well to be happy," or "think well to be healthy." It now also means "think well to be happIER," and "think well to be healthIER," and "think well to be mentally okay," and "think well to find balance," and "think well to retrain your brain," and "think well to... get to neutral." ☺ (Thank you, Grandpa Alan.)

I am passionate about sharing what I've been taught and helping others learn the tools to feel more control over their well-being. So, turn the page, and let's get started.

PART 1

WHY SHOULD
WE STRESS LESS?

1

MINDFULNESS MATTERS

The Importance of the Present

As a teen myself, I know that the stress and emotions that come with this time in our lives can sometimes feel overwhelming. But we have to remember that we are not alone. We're not exactly alike, but we have all felt joy, anxiety, depression and so many other feelings.

When I first started advocating for mental health awareness, I was concerned that I wasn't going to be able to make a big enough impact because the statistics were so high – and so scary. Mental health issues like anxiety, depression, bullying and anger – and the possible outcomes of mental health conditions, such as suicide and homicide – have doubled among kids and teens in the past few years. Suicide is the second most common cause of death among young people in the US; at the time I'm writing this, that's 45,000 people a year. Seventy percent of teens, according to *The New York Times*, say mental health issues are the number one problem they face.[1]

What can we do to make things better? We need the right tools to handle these rough times, and we need to practice them every day, even when we feel our best, so that we're prepared to face the moments when we feel our worst.

WHAT IS MINDFULNESS?

There are a lot of definitions floating around, but the one I like best is that *mindfulness is focusing on the moment we're in without judgment, not worrying about yesterday or tomorrow.* So, it's the ability to notice what's happening right now and not get overwhelmed by what's going on around us, what has already happened or what hasn't happened yet.

Mindfulness is *not* about stopping all negative thoughts because that's not realistic. It's about knowing that we can acknowledge those thoughts, then release them. We have the power over how much we want to focus on a thought or event; thoughts don't control or define us. We can make a choice not to worry and to instead be happier and healthier right now, in this moment. And, if we can pay attention to the present moment, we can live in kindness toward ourselves and others.

Embracing mindfulness practices has helped me get through the ups and downs of teenage life, and it can help you too. We can learn to cope with stress and emotions in a healthier way. Through my work with Wuf Shanti, I have found that kids can be taught mindfulness at an early age, which allows them to grow up to be happier, more empathetic adults, and deal with whatever life throws at them in a more productive manner. Having healthy coping mechanisms can also help us overcome anxiety, cultivate a more positive mindset, dissolve negative thoughts and make better decisions on the path to achieving our goals.

SHOW ME THE SCIENCE

Lots of people ask me why they should care about mindfulness. Pediatrician Dr. Dzung Vo told me, "There's a lot of science behind mindfulness. It affects your body, physiology, blood pressure, the way your brain functions… You can see how mindfulness affects your own breathing or heart rate or muscle tension." And it's true! In fact, there are thousands of scientific studies showing the benefits of practicing mindfulness (including improvements in physical health, mental health, learning, athletics and more).

HOW CAN MINDFULNESS HELP ME?

Mentally and emotionally, mindfulness helps enhance:

- Focus
- Understanding
- Tolerance
- Emotional intelligence
- Self-esteem
- Self-confidence
- Self-acceptance
- Self-compassion
- Kindness
- Gratitude
- Connection
- Compassion
- Memory
- Mood
- Empathy.

Physically, mindfulness improves:

- Immunity
- Respiration
- Digestion
- Blood pressure
- Cardiovascular fitness
- Bone strength
- Muscle and joint strength
- Energy

- Flexibility
- Endurance
- Balance
- Core strength
- Posture
- Sleep.

You may be thinking, "*Yeah, right, how can this one thing do all of that?*" Or maybe you're thinking, "*Ugh, I don't have time for this,*" or, "*I don't want to have to do something boring with my time,*" but practicing mindfulness to get those results doesn't have to be boring, and it can be done in a few minutes, at any time of day. Okay, so maybe now you're thinking, "*But I'm not doing any of that weird stuff!*"

WHAT DOES "BEING MINDFUL" LOOK LIKE?

Mindfulness is *not* about sitting with your eyes closed, your legs crossed and your hands making the "OK" sign on your knees, and it is way more than just breathing… although breathing is kind of important, right? (Lol, I laughed). As mindfulness author Whitney Stewart puts it, "Mindfulness includes a conversation with students and talking with them about the conflicts they face and challenges they have and finding ways they can work through those social and emotional difficulties, not just sitting and breathing mindfully before class."

You can practice mindfulness in any way that is comfortable to you, and we'll explore many potential methods for doing so in **Part 2**. For now, let's focus on one of the most integral elements of mindfulness: learning not to give power to the negative loop in our heads. The goal is simply to focus on something other than your negative thoughts, and if your mind wanders, to learn how to bring it back.

Even my little sister, when she was around four years old, figured out how to do it. One day, I heard her controlling her own temper tantrum. She was upset about something – I don't remember what – and all of a sudden, she started tapping her fingers together and repeating, "Peace begins with me," and, "Think well to be well." To our surprise, this four-year-old child used mantras to get her emotions under control.

Have you ever had one of those days where everything seems to be going wrong? It happens to everyone, including me. Well, there are really only three things you can do when that happens: laugh, cry or breathe. We've all been taught that we have a choice to make: We can see the glass half full, or we can see it as half empty. But are those really the only choices? Isn't the cup refillable? That's a really powerful thought to consider because it means that we can always rewire our brains. We just have to practice refilling our cup!

It takes lots of mindfulness practice to get to this place of optimism. But getting there means that when stressful things happen – *and they will* – you'll already have the tools to help you deal with them. If you practice and learn to be present, it can lead to gratitude, self-love and self-compassion. Think of it as the ultimate form of self-care. Using just one mindfulness practice can keep you from slipping down a rabbit hole. You may find it keeps you from being stuck in the sadness of yesterday or the anxiety of tomorrow.

> Dave Smith of the Secular Dharma Foundation shared with me that he suffered intensely as a teenager, feeling like he didn't fit in or have any friends – but mindfulness changed his perspective.
>
> He said, "Mindfulness saved my life. It allowed me to realize there were things I could do in terms of what I thought about life, and that was a tremendous relief. It's the most basic skills of mindfulness that are important. If you

can't dribble a ball, you can't play basketball. Learning that I could pay attention to something other than what I was thinking about blew my mind. I learned that I could get out of my mind and the story going on inside of it. Now, I have a 'check engine' light that goes on when I'm feeling angry, scared or sad, and instead of freaking out, I relax and take a deep breath because I've trained my mind to do that."

My friend, Andrew, a junior in high school, was very stressed out all the time and overwhelmed, always in a bad mood, and everything was so serious to him. After he learned mindfulness, his whole demeanor changed. He smiled more, cracked jokes and didn't get angry as often – all because he learned to use mindfulness to cope with his stress and emotions. It literally took him a few minutes each day.

To watch my friend become happier and less stressed made me happy too. The fact that something I believe in helped one person, especially someone I care about, made me feel like I would be able to make an impact.

As you know, there are lots of mindfulness techniques in this book. Find which ones you like and make them part of your daily routine. Like Dave and Andrew, you may just find that you're better prepared to face all the ups and downs of life with a few mindful practices in your back pocket.

JOURNALING BREAK:
Mindfulness, focus and taking a pause

- What is mindfulness to you?
  - What distracts you?
  - What makes your mind wander to yesterday or tomorrow?
- How do you usually make yourself focus?
  - When you are really focused on something, do you find that your mind still wanders?
  - How do you feel when you're in the present moment?
- Have you ever felt upset and paused for a few seconds or taken a breath before replying? Did it make you feel more in control of your emotions?

2

REWIRING THE BRAIN

The Power of SEL

As you get older, your brain continues to develop, all the way through our teen years and beyond. You form habits in how you speak to yourself, how you care for your body and mind, and how you get along with others. However, no matter how old you get, you *can* change.

We all have the power to re-train our brains, and with a little practice, we can actually achieve two things that can transform our sense of well-being: **choice** and **control**. We are bombarded with a multitude of messages every day, from teachers, parents, friends, celebrities, television, social media and more. And, unless we are taught otherwise, teens tend to focus on the negative messages we receive, which have more of a lasting impact on our minds.

WHAT IS SEL?

Social-emotional learning (SEL) is the process of developing the self-awareness, self-regulation and interpersonal skills that are so essential in life. If you can recognize, understand and accept your emotions, then you can learn appropriate ways to respond to them, and this, in turn, will help you build better relationships with yourselves and others. SEL teaches you to cope with stress and emotions, and show self-compassion and resilience, all of which is empowering because it means that no one controls your reactions other than you.

SEL doesn't demand that you're happy 100 percent of the time, but it does help you get to a more positive place – or at least to a neutral place. By learning the tools to help you feel happier and healthier, you can reduce self-harm and harm to others. Communication, connection, interaction with others and collaboration are also vital SEL skills.

> **"The skills learned in school are what you will need when you're in the workforce... you need it in today's world."**
>
> **– Tim Ryan, former US Congressman**
>
> The above quote comes from a conversation I had with former US Congressman Tim Ryan, and I completely agree with him. One of my jobs was at a cookie store (the best cookies ever, btw!), and my boss felt very strongly about the hospitality culture – about how we interacted with our customers and made sure they had a great experience that contributed to them having a great day. In fact, before anyone could become a full-time employee, he required them to read a book about hospitality, which had a lot of SEL principles in it, and then he sat down with each person one on one to discuss what was learned. This was far more meaningful to him than whether we knew how to use the cash register or not.

> **"If you really want to reach peace, then begin by educating the children."**
>
> **– Gandhi**
>
> Learning how to treat ourselves and get along with others matters just as much as learning to read and write, so classes in emotional healing and interacting with others should be incorporated into schools. That may be a controversial thing to say, but I don't know how we can expect kids to grow into productive and empathetic teens and adults if we don't teach them how to be.

INVEST IN YOURSELF

Psychologist Dr. Rick Hanson says, "The social-emotional skills of mindfulness are the most important things to learn because you can apply that to anything you want to grow inside. Realize investing in yourself is a really smart thing to do in the long term even if it's a pain for a few years when you're young."

Inner peace may be a difficult concept to wrap your head around, but it's something that is actually attainable – with practice. Learning more about yourself, how you handle situational stress and how you navigate your way through life are key skills to learn. Think how much easier and potentially happier your adult life will be if you figure this out now.

This is why there is a such a big push, supported by the Collaborative for Academic, Social and Emotional Learning (CASEL), to get these programs into our education system. CASEL's Heather Schwartz defines SEL as "how we learn to get along with people who are different from us, handle stress, collaborate with others, understand our own emotions, and the environments in which we do these things, and learning experiences that connect the head and the heart." She goes on to say, "The majority of SEL programs include some mindfulness that includes the ability to stop and take a moment. In order for us to make choices and use the skills we've learned, we have to be able to pause."

> **"Life moves pretty fast. If you don't stop and look around once in a while, you could miss it."**
> *– Ferris Bueller's Day Off*

MINDFULNESS AND SEL

Can we have mindfulness without SEL and vice versa? In my mind, they are linked. And, according to Laura Bakosh, "Mindfulness-based social-emotional learning (MBSEL) is considered 'next-generation SEL' because it addresses the roots of underperformance and 'diseases of despair' (depression, violence, addiction, suicide, self-harm) by reducing stress and priming the intellect for learning."

MBSEL tools are essential life skills. In my TEDx Talk, I said that it's crucial to learn mindfulness and social-emotional learning in addition to traditional academic subjects. Mindfulness, social-emotional learning and emotional intelligence are mandatory coursework in other countries, and I believe that they should be part of the core curriculum in American schools too. These tools are necessary to get a good job, keep a good job, be happy, healthy – and to navigate life. We need to be able to know and understand how we're feeling and be able to cope and respond in appropriate ways; to know we have support systems and learn to communicate with each other so we can build resilience and bounce back; to ask more questions of ourselves and others; and put ourselves in other people's shoes to gain compassion and empathy.[2]

Maybe you're thinking, "*Okay, but that's easier said than done. It's not so easy to change the way I've been dealing with my stress and emotions or interacting with others."* I get it, believe me – it's even hard for me sometimes to cope with stress or put my phone down. But it is possible to learn these skills. There are a lot of practices that can help us handle emotions, enjoy life and laugh more. I believe these are the skills we need to be taught to get there:

HOW TO SPEAK, RESPECT AND APPRECIATE DIFFERENCES, AND BE KIND TO YOURSELF AND OTHERS

I don't know about you, but I'm tired of turning on the TV and seeing the same stuff on the news about bullying, depression and violence. There are more incidences of bullying (one in five kids is bullied), isolation, suicide and homicide in kids and teens under 18 than ever before. Whether it's due to cellphones, social media, video games or how society is today doesn't matter – there is a mental health crisis in our country. Pre-teens and teens in middle school spend around eight hours in front of media every day, which may lead to increased aggressiveness, desensitization and lower self-esteem.[3]

Instead, teens need to be taught how to speak with each other, respect and appreciate differences, and be kind to themselves and each other. Developing values, empathy and skills to manage relationships helps you develop socially. And all of these skills help you in learning how to cope with stress, anger, anxiety and depression; manage your behavior by self-regulating; and resolve conflict by making smart choices.

HOW TO CONVEY THOUGHTS EFFECTIVELY AND BE AWARE OF THE WORLD AROUND YOU

Once you learn how to communicate with others and express yourself, then you can learn compassion. If everyone does the same, then we can begin to heal this planet. One way to raise your awareness is through pro-social behavior, such as sharing, volunteering or donating. Doing so teaches you to be trustworthy, helpful, kind and take other views into account – all of which will serve you well in adulthood.

HOW TO HANDLE STRESS AND ANGER IN A CALM AND PEACEFUL WAY

Life is busy, fast paced and complicated, so in order to navigate strong emotions, lower self-harm rates and harm to others, it's important to focus on well-being, self-awareness, social skills, empathy and self-management. Learning to solve problems in healthy ways – without violence or trauma – is vital, too. Stress impairs learning, but regulating thoughts and emotions, communicating mindfully, and focusing on the now, helps you pay greater attention and do better in school academically and behaviorally.

I've seen through my work with Wuf Shanti that kids can learn to think positively, appreciate what is good and spread love and peace, helping them to become more self-aware, empathetic, kind and focused. That's why I believe that MBSEL curriculum is crucial for teens to learn appropriate responsive behavior so we can self-correct, be our authentic selves, build trust, become less obsessed with the past and future, and experience an increase in happiness. Our brains may still be developing every day, and we might be changing, but by learning MBSEL practices, we'll gain control and choice over our emotions.

JOURNALING BREAK:
Solving a stressor

1. Write a list of ten things that stress you out.
2. Next to each stressor, write the word "temporary" or "permanent"; then, decide and write down if the stressor is "in your control" or "out of your control."
3. For the ones that you can't control, cross them out.
4. What's left are the ones that you can work on. Pick one of those and write potential steps for finding the solution.

3

FINDING "ME"

Focusing on the Self

How can you be happy? Under the theory of positive psychology – the study of how we can thrive and live a fulfilling life – MBSEL stands out as one of our most useful tools. As positive-psychology author Dr. Diane Gehart puts it, "Understanding what makes us happy is more than a luxury right now, and it's a very serious topic. If the only time you're happy is when someone else is telling you that 'you are okay, you're good enough,' then you're going to have a very unstable sense of happiness."

CASEL has detailed the five components of an SEL-based curriculum that can help us understand and manage our emotions. They are:

- Self-awareness
- Self-management
- Social awareness
- Relationship skills
- Responsible decision-making.

Because we are focusing on the self – you – in this chapter, we're going to talk about three of them: self-awareness and self-management, as well as responsible decision-making, which is linked to all five components of finding happiness.

SELF-AWARENESS

According to CASEL, "Self-awareness is the ability to understand one's own emotions, thoughts and values, and how they influence behavior across contexts, including the capacity to recognize one's strengths and limitations with a well-grounded sense of confidence and purpose."[4]

This means that you have to become good at naming your feelings and talking about them, like an internal conversation with yourself. We all have to ask ourselves questions, like "How am *I* doing?" and listen to the answers in an honest way, with integrity. Dave Smith said, "Most people, if they are angry, think about blaming someone. The key is to create a choice point. We get to choose what we do. Mindfulness plus choice is freedom." Emotional intelligence (EI) expert and host of Parent-TV Supna Shah agrees. She says, "What we do with our emotions is our choice. It's what makes us human." It means you're able to recognize and understand the emotion that you're feeling while you're feeling it. For some people, that's not an easy task, but it can be learned.

A friend of mine, Skylar, was always a super serious person. She would rarely just let go and laugh – it seemed like she was always carrying the weight of the world on her shoulders.

One day I asked her what was going on, and whether there was anything I could do to help. She started telling me about how she has so many family responsibilities, and she gets angry and resentful when she sees her siblings living a carefree, happy – and what she described as selfish – life. It was eating her up inside. Once she said out loud how she was feeling, I think she was able to accept that the way they lived their lives was not the cause of her anger. Her feelings were a choice that she was making. I described to her a practice that she could try, and it's one that you might want to try, too:

Look in the mirror and repeat a positive affirmation, such as, "I am worthy of laughter, love and joy." (I'll share a lot more positive affirmation ideas in Chapter 10.)

Later that week, I saw Skylar laughing with some of our friends. I'm glad she found a practice that worked for her. Since then, Skylar has come to a place of self-acceptance by checking in with herself and realizing that it is okay to feel her emotions.

Once you understand how you're feeling, you can identify your self-talk habits and develop new ones that can raise your self-confidence and self-esteem levels. Strong emotions can cloud your ability to make healthy choices, so if you understand how to process them, then that directly correlates with making better choices. As Maureik Robison of Inner Explorer explains, we have a choice as to how we handle a situation. He says, "A reaction is mind*less*, and a response is mindful. To do anything well, you first have to have an awareness of what you're doing."

When I'm under a lot of stress, whether it's from having too much homework, not feeling well or even when my basketball team, the Miami HEAT, are in a close game in the fourth quarter (just ask my friends!), I first have to check in with myself to uncover how I'm feeling. I'll take some deep breaths and figure out whether I'm jumping to blame someone or something for my mental state, and how to best express my emotions. I've reacted and yelled out of frustration before, sure, but that didn't help my situation or make me feel any better. I try to remember that and respond differently now.

It may seem easy to recognize anger, sadness and worry, but is it easy to understand how your body feels when you're angry, what happens to your breath and your brain when you worry, and how emotions affect your interactions with others? You might be thinking, "No, it's not," but your answer can change with the help of self-awareness. Feelings are transient – they come and go and change, and so does their intensity. Mindfully observing and listening to yourself and others builds focus and attention skills.

Self-compassion author Karen Bluth urges teens to "be yourselves, and know that you are a wonderful, terrific person just as you are. You may not believe that right now in this moment, but just be open to the possibility of that maybe being true." When you identify and accept your feelings, then you're on the road to healing and authenticity. With self-awareness, you can learn that being imperfect is perfect.

So, how do you become aware of how you are feeling, understand those feelings and pay attention to them with kindness? These practices can help:

SELF-AWARENESS PRACTICE:
Mirroring

- Look in the mirror and see how your face and body look when you are happy/angry/sad.
- Pay attention to how your body feels by listening to it.
- Or, you can also ask a friend or family member to be the mirror and reflect your emotions back to you.
- Watch and listen, and notice how their changes in demeanor make you feel.
- Then, switch places, and they will be the emotions, and you can be the mirror.

SELF-AWARENESS PRACTICE:
Lists

You can learn to focus mindfully by making lists, whether they're in your head or physically written down. Create any one of the following lists to boost your self-awareness:

- Check in with your senses – what can you see, hear, etc.?
- Consider cause and effect – what causes you to feel angry, or what is the effect of feeling angry?
- Think about your goals and dreams – what do you want, and what will it take to get there?
- Think about your most special qualities, including personal and cultural assets, to remind yourself of all you have to offer. (You'll practice this one in the JOURNALING BREAK for this section.)
- Examine your prejudices and biases to help yourself let go of them.
- Write down when you are sad or upset to become aware of what causes those emotions and how your body and mind react to them.

SELF-AWARENESS PRACTICE:
Affirmations

Affirmations are an amazing and effective way to address negative self-talk. In the second part of this book, I include a specific affirmation practice on page 115 with some of my favorite affirmations to repeat when I need positive reinforcement.

JOURNALING BREAK:
Talents and limiting beliefs

- We all have talents, something we're good at, such as being kind, playing sports, doing art, singing. What are you good at? What do you like about yourself? Make a list of at least three qualities and talents that you have.

- How does it make you feel when people give you compliments?
- Write down two or three limiting beliefs you have, such as, "I am not good enough," or "I am not lovable." Then, reverse the belief, and write the opposite: "I AM good enough," or "I AM lovable." (Pro tip: You can then use your reverse beliefs as positive affirmations!)
- Write down the top ten most important things in your life, then rank them in order of importance. Finally, assign a percentage to the amount of time you give to each of those things. Do they match? If not, how can you change that?

Remember: Emotions can be strong, overpowering and confusing. But once you begin to name and own your feelings, you can move on to learning how to manage them.

SELF-MANAGEMENT

According to CASEL, "Self-management is the ability to manage one's emotions, thoughts and behaviors effectively in different situations and to achieve goals and aspirations, including the capacity to delay gratification, manage stress and feel motivation and agency to accomplish personal and collective goals."[5]

I interpret it as self-regulation, meaning that we can figure out how to deal with our emotions by learning:

- Positive self-talk habits
- Calming techniques

- Optimism
- Self-control
- How to pause to stop impulsive behavior.

Self-regulation revolves around the understanding that your body and brain are connected (for example, how your heart rate goes up or your breathing gets fast when you're upset) and why that matters (because your brain and your organs are not getting enough oxygen). Only then can you begin to understand why coping with and releasing those emotions in an appropriate way can allow you to live a healthier life.

None of this happens overnight though. I still let my emotions get the best of me sometimes. Having a growth mindset means that it's okay to make mistakes because you're learning, and struggles make you stronger. I like to teach students about grit and "the power of yet." The power of yet means that you can rethink something in a more positive way, giving yourself some grace. For example, "I don't understand how to get from anger to joy," can be "I don't understand how to get from anger to joy **yet**." Have patience with yourself because you will get it if you keep practicing.

Casey is a friend of mine whose brother died by suicide. Casey, understandably, was having trouble dealing with the loss. They were sad and angry. At first, they isolated and stopped talking to their friends. But then, Casey started to journal and find a passion for music, and through these outlets, they were able to process the emotions and start opening the lines of communication again.

This process wasn't easy or fast for Casey – it isn't for any of us. The goals you set for yourself need to be realistic so that you can self-motivate. You should also give yourself a pat on the back when you've achieved something.

Remember, too, that people have lots of different ways for processing, regulating and releasing their emotions. Sadiqa Glusman, formerly of Heal the Planet, said that when she's angry, she puts on comedy, which makes her feel better in the moment and helps her find a positive way to cope. She said laughter brings her out of the past and future, and helps her be fully present in the now. Anger is a particularly hard emotion to deal with, but you learn perseverance through challenges, and you gain self-compassion and compassion for others in the process.

JOURNALING BREAK:
Learning to handle emotions

- What does "respond instead of react" mean to you? Think of a situation where you instantly reacted and regretted it. How could pausing before responding have helped you in that situation?
- What does the term "temporary" mean to you? How can you use this definition to help you through difficult emotions?
- What does "being assertive" mean to you? Do you think you can be assertive without being rude, dismissive or aggressive? How?
- Make a list of up to five negative thoughts that you had today. Then, change them into positive thoughts. For example, change "I can't" to "I can," "I'm not" to "I am," etc.

When stress gets out of control, it can have a negative effect on your physical and mental health and wellness – as I said before, the brain and body are connected, and recognizing this is key to self-management.

SELF-MANAGEMENT PRACTICE:
Stress reduction

As you have probably started to notice, there are a lot of stress-reduction practices in this book, and you can choose any one of them to help you with self-regulation. But while we're on the subject, here are a few ways to hone your stress-reduction and stress-management skills:

- Create checklists for goals to track and see progress along the way.
- Write down how things could have gone worse in a situation that's causing you stress.
- Brainstorm positive ways to manage sadness, anger and anxiety. For example:
  - List ways to show yourself care (whether it's through hobbies you enjoy, sports you play, music you like, etc.)
  - Visualize how you might handle situations differently.
  - Role-play – based on hypotheticals or what's happening to you in real life – to practice how to respond instead of reacting.

Knowing how to be less stressed is a gift to ourselves. Yes, it takes a few minutes every day, but practicing these techniques can literally change the brain, creating habitual positive behaviors. If you don't do something about your internal stress, it can lead to longer-lasting mental health conditions, which is why stress reduction and self-regulation are so important to learn now. You can choose how to act, you can think before you speak, you can decide whether to accept or judge, and you can live in gratitude. All these choices help you toward getting along better with yourself and others, and help you learn how to be happier – and a lot less stressed.

RESPONSIBLE DECISION-MAKING

According to CASEL, "Responsible decision-making is the ability to make caring and constructive choices about personal behavior and social interactions across diverse situations, including the capacity to consider ethical standards and safety concerns, and to evaluate the benefits and consequences of various actions for personal, social and collective well-being."[6]

Part of decision-making is identifying goals and the steps required to reach those goals, and to make conscious choices, we need to first be able to analyze information, and anticipate, evaluate and appreciate rules and the consequences of our actions. While problem-solving is a skill we learn when we're young, as we grow up and the conflicts become bigger, we need to be able to identify and clearly articulate alternative solutions and know when to get help.

JOURNALING BREAK:
Goals

- Write three to five specific, attainable goals that you have for yourself, and then explain why each one is important to you.
- Write down the tasks that it will take to achieve those goals. Create a timeline for achieving each goal.

When my grandpa sat me down to talk about the rules for driving, the number one rule was not to drink and drive, nor to get into the car with anyone who was impaired by any kind of substance. At the time, I rolled my eyes and said, "Duh." I thought to myself, *"Who in their right mind would ever do something like that?"* Then, I had to check myself, because there are a lot of people who would make a different decision than I would, not only in that circumstance, but in many other situations as well.

JOURNALING BREAK:
Responsible decision-making in practice

- How do you usually make decisions? Do you think about them really hard? Or do you just make really fast decisions based on what your intuition tells you?
  - How do you think your decision-making style hurts or helps you?
- Do you apply ethical reasoning in your own decisions? Think about the following situations. How – and what – would you decide to do in each one?
  - Someone offers you alcohol or drugs.
  - A friend wants you to get in the car with someone who has been drinking.
  - Bullies urge you to join them in teasing your friend.
  - Classmates want you to join in defacing school property.
  - A friend tries to get you to blow off studying for a test.
  - You are in an argument with your parents and have the urge to say something disrespectful.
- Write about a time that you made a choice based on a strong emotion, and how you felt about that choice

once the anger subsided. In hindsight, should you have handled it differently? What would have been the responsible way to make your decision?

We each have innate goodness, and recognizing that is key to becoming our best selves, shifting away from destructive behaviors and focusing our attention on the positive. Sometimes, it's hard to be open-minded, but by implementing critical-thinking skills, you can begin to reflect on how your decisions affect your well-being and the well-being of others.

How to practice decision-making skills:

- Think of hypothetical scenarios or dialogues to demonstrate inappropriate and appropriate ways to handle situations.
- Brainstorm positive ways to solve problems, or ways to be a buddy and help someone who is being teased.
- Choose to spend time with people who build you up.

The future holds so many possibilities, and you can make healthier choices and celebrate small accomplishments by saying nice things to yourself, believing in yourself, finding a way to contribute to society and feeling hopeful for making a positive difference.

Of course, as you grow up, your purpose can and will likely change as you evolve, but part of making responsible decisions is figuring out how to resolve challenges without giving up pursuit of our goal. As Winston Churchill said, we should "never,

ever, ever quit." If we make a goal, we should try to stick to it. Or, as Yoda says in *Star Wars Episode V: The Empire Strikes Back*, "Do or do not. There is no try." In other words, if it doesn't work the first time, go another route. Believe in yourself and keep going, with every bit of determination you can muster.

4

UNDERSTANDING US

... and Considering Others

I never said that figuring out how to do all this is easy, but it is doable, especially if you start practicing early. It's a toss-up as to which is more difficult: knowing and accepting emotions within yourself, or understanding where others are coming from and how to connect on an authentic level.

SOCIAL AWARENESS

As CASEL puts it, "Social awareness is the ability to understand the perspectives of and empathize with others, including those from diverse backgrounds, cultures and contexts."[7]

Self-awareness and self-regulation – which we just discussed in Chapter 3 – allow you to be your true self and accept that you're worthy of love and kindness. With social awareness, you will learn to:

- Understand how other people feel
- Recognize strengths in others
- Show concern for the feelings of others
- Interact with others.

How you interact with people, how you affect them and how they affect you – these are the central steps to becoming socially aware.

You can't assume that everyone thinks the same or feels the same as you do. People think and feel differently, so it's vital to practice seeing different perspectives and points of view. Because of your individual background and culture, you may not relate to something that would upset someone from a different walk of life in a given situation or event. The only way to become aware of other people's feelings is to try to put yourself in their shoes so that you can be more understanding, compassionate and empathetic. You can learn to predict feelings and recognize non-verbal cues, such as facial expressions and body language. You can notice how kindness makes you feel, and how it makes others feel. And you can learn how to be grateful and express that gratitude.

> During the Covid-19 pandemic, I (and so many others around the world) learned to be grateful for things that we had previously taken for granted. I could have been miserable every day – and made others miserable as well – but I instead faced the Covid challenge with a positive mindset, understanding that opportunities exist in every situation. I made a conscious effort to see what possibilities existed, and I used the time to write this book.

In virtually any situation, something good can be derived from something negative. Everyone gets frustrated sometimes – with themselves and their circumstances, or with something that another person says or does – but you need to be patient and try to find the positive. I remember when the late Jane Marczewski, a contestant on *America's Got Talent* who was battling cancer, said, "We can't wait until life isn't hard before we decide to be happy."

If Jane found the positive, you can too. It only takes a willingness to learn. You can show people that you appreciate them by:

- Listening and speaking with kindness
- Asking more questions
- Understanding individual and group differences
- Working through challenges together
- Appreciating positive influences
- Showing concern and helping them when you can.

Social awareness is about appreciating diversity and inclusion, valuing other perspectives and understanding that everyone's feelings are valid, all while being your authentic self. With everything going on in the world, social awareness is more essential than ever.

It's okay if you don't get it right away. Remember that setbacks are temporary, and mistakes are opportunities to learn. And you have family, school and community support to help you along the way. As Dr. Amy Saltzman, author of *A Still Quiet Place*, says, "As teens and human beings, we can spend a lot of time beating ourselves up, so it's really important to pay attention with kindness and compassion and a sense of humor so that we can change our behavior." I think that's true. We have to give ourselves a break, and as long as we have the best of intentions, we will ultimately succeed in sending kindness and compassion to ourselves and others.

JOURNALING BREAK:
Compassion

- What does compassion mean to you? Is there a difference between compassion and empathy?
- Do you find it easy to forgive and forget? Why or why not?

- Think back on a difficult time in your life. How did others show you compassion? List the ways they did, and then describe how one such effort made you feel.
  - How can you be compassionate when others face similar situations?

How to improve social awareness:

- Practice giving and receiving compliments.
- Notice the similarities and differences between yourself and a friend or classmate.
- Consider the importance of attentiveness and, alternatively, how it feels to be ignored or feel invisible.
- Write a poem about being a good friend or community member.
- Think about how a new student may feel and come up with a list of ways to help them.
- Write about a time you saw someone being mistreated or left out and how that person probably felt.
- Role-play how you'd feel in someone else's shoes in a particular situation, imagining their perspective and how you might help that person.
- Role-play being an upstander – someone who takes a stand for a positive cause – to develop pro-social behavior.
- List the ways that people showed you compassion during difficult times.
- Develop a service project to help the community.
- Interview a peer about character traits.

RELATIONSHIP SKILLS

Once you understand how others feel, and how that affects you, you need to bring your attention to how you interact with a diverse group of people. According to CASEL, "Relationship skills are the ability to establish and maintain healthy and supportive relationships and to effectively navigate settings with diverse individuals and groups."[8]

Think about it this way: When your parents or friends annoy you, are you calm and able to interact with kindness toward them, and vice versa? I don't think anyone would say that it's possible to always communicate effectively or get along with everyone. That's because verbal and non-verbal cues can result in misunderstandings or hurt feelings.

I once got into an argument via text with a friend about a political issue (which I won't go into here because it's not the focus of the story – suffice it to say that it was a controversial topic). We were sending messages back and forth and getting upset, as each of us was passionate about our viewpoints.

I ended up calling my friend, and we spoke on the phone to make sure we both felt heard. Even though we ultimately disagreed, it was important to look at each other's perspectives from our different cultures and the way we were raised, the history of our people and the way the world is now.

Sometimes it's hard to remove all the noise, but if you take a step back, you can see the bigger picture and engage in a respectful discussion.

JOURNALING BREAK:
Friendship

- What does "BFF" mean to you?
- Can you be your own BFF? How?
- What qualities would you like to have in a friend?
  - After writing them down, think about your close friends. Do they embody the qualities you listed? If not, how can you connect with people who do?
  - Now, think about yourself as a friend. Do you embody the qualities you listed? How can you improve?
- How did you feel when you hear your friends say nice things about you?
- How do you feel when you say kind words about your friends? How do you think it makes them feel?

We can learn positive communication skills to help us forge and maintain healthy relationships. After all, the keys to building lasting positive relationships are:

- Communication
- Compassion
- Connection.

> **"Forgive yourself for not knowing what you didn't before you learned it."**
>
> **– Maya Angelou**

Positive communication can help us show compassion and build connections, too. For example, if everyone used "I" statements in disagreements (as opposed to statements that start with "you," which may make someone feel blamed or misunderstood), it would avoid a lot of arguments. "I" statements are just one way to de-escalate potential conflicts – using non-inflammatory language, holding eye contact and using a kind tone of voice will also work. Some things are a little harder, like patience and forgiveness, but they're achievable with active listening and attentive focus. And don't be afraid to make mistakes – as Maya Angelou once said, "Forgive yourself for not knowing what you didn't know before you learned it."[9]

> If my parents and I disagree on something, I try to remember that they are coming at it from a different perspective and have the best of intentions. Pausing to reflect on that usually stops me from snapping at them – notice how I didn't say "always"! Sometimes it's hard to engage in dialogue with love and respect, like when you're in a bad mood and what you say doesn't come out the way you intended it to sound. Mindfulness and SEL help us think before we speak and allow us the space to make kinder choices.

JOURNALING BREAK:
De-escalating conflict

- Write about how you would handle each of these situations, and how you would communicate your displeasure in a kind way:
  - You are mad that your friend is spending more time with someone else.
  - You are scared about Covid and want to make sure your family is safe.
  - Your teacher tells you that they think you are not doing your best in class.

- You are overwhelmed when your parents ask you to watch your younger sibling because you have a ton of homework.
- Someone you know is making fun of another person or being mean to them.

More ways to learn relationship skills:

- Play games that require taking turns.
- Pass a ball to practice conversation skills.
- Try team-building exercises or virtual relay games for learning cooperation.
- Role-play
  - How to solve conflicts.
  - Polite ways to talk about difficult conversations, offering support or help when needed.
- Practice eye contact while a person talks to demonstrate attention and respect.
- Practice your tone of voice in conversations.
- Speak to a classmate or friend, then paraphrase what your partner says to practice good listening skills.
- Write gratitude notes.
- Write about a time you had to cooperate with someone to get something done.

COMMUNITY

To be part of a community means thinking of others before we say or do things, and responding to their emotions in a respectful way. Teens have the added pressure of dealing with social media communities, too. We need to figure out how to post and talk online consciously, which means pausing before we post.

In all these situations, you can acknowledge how people feel without agreeing with them, and you can learn how to de-escalate conflict or resolve a problem before it becomes a bigger problem by gaining self-control and slowing down, pausing and listening, and breathing. Remember to try and exhibit positive behavior, too, because other people are watching and learning from you.

As a leader aiming to make a positive impact, I model the behavior I'd like to see from others. Even if it's something as simple as turning off my phone instead of reacting to something that upsets me or with which I disagree, I do what I can to regain balance and perspective. I always think, if someone sees me interacting with kindness, being an upstander to stick up for others and using my voice for good, maybe they will do the same, and then someone else will notice, and so on.

JOURNALING BREAK:
Cooperation

- What does cooperation mean to you?
- Do you like working on projects with others? Why or why not?
- Have you ever had a disagreement with a friend while you were working together on a project? How did you resolve it?
- What does it mean to be part of a team?
- What kind of things do you think need to be addressed within your community? How would you resolve those issues?
- Develop a service project to help the community.

- ○ Who would you help?
- ○ How would you help them?
- ○ How does this benefit the community?
- ○ What are your action steps?
- How does it make you feel to help others?

5

GIVING YOURSELF A BREAK

Gaining Strength, Self-Compassion and Resilience

Let's recap everything you've learned so far: understanding your feelings, expressing your feelings, understanding other people's feelings and interacting with people in your community. All together, these components contribute to your development of acceptance, self-compassion, resilience and empathy for others. They may not be listed along with the CASEL components I shared in Chapters 3 and 4, but both self-compassion and resilience are directly intertwined with MBSEL.

> **"You want to focus on the relationship with yourself because that's the relationship that you're going to have for your whole life."**
>
> **– Dave Smith**

SELF-COMPASSION

Dave Smith says, "Teenagers are tremendously hard on themselves. That's where your power lies. Kindness starts with you. Are you kind to yourself when you make a mistake? Are you grateful to yourself when you do well, get a good grade, or your sports team does well? You want to focus on the relationship with yourself because that's the relationship that you're going to have for your whole life." Getting to a place of self-compassion makes it a whole lot easier to gain compassion for others.

Life happens – sometimes it's great, and sometimes it's frustrating. Our challenge is figuring out the best way to maneuver the ups and downs. Todd Wolfenberg of Yoga International says, "We're going to have good days and bad days, happiness and depressions, and that's okay. Honesty and openness about that really helps the process." Even when awful things happen or you have a hard day, you need to be compassionate with yourself and others, because you have no idea what's going on in their lives.

SELF-COMPASSION PRACTICE:
Kind words and kind beings

1. Speak kind words to yourself. Look in the mirror at yourself and say things like:
   - "I love you."
   - "I am nice."
   - "I am kind."
   - "I am friendly".
   … or any other positive feedback you have for yourself.
2. Picture yourself surrounded by kind beings who are sending you love and goodwill. Imagine yourself sending the same love and goodwill to others.

JOURNALING BREAK:
Self-compassion

- What does self-compassion mean to you?
- How can we show ourselves compassion?

- Do you treat yourself better than others, or do you treat others better than yourself? Why?
- Write yourself a letter as if you were talking to your best friend in the world, from the compassionate part of yourself to the part of yourself that is struggling. What would you say to your best friend – in this case, yourself?

RESILIENCE

Jessica Morey of Inward Bound Mindfulness Education says, "There's so much happening in the world, like *big* issues... Mindful compassion practices can help us build resilience, so when things get really tough, we have the internal resources to not freak out. It can help us have enough space to decide a skillful way of responding."

Resilience is a hard concept – I struggled with it initially, too. Intellectually, I understood that it means that we face challenges and bounce back from problems. German philosopher Friedrich Nietzsche said, "That which does not kill us, makes us stronger," [and so did Kelly Clarkson in her song, "Stronger (What Doesn't Kill You)."][10] And as Dave Smith explains, "Resilience is the ability to overcome a challenge... Stress is a perception or an idea that we don't have the internal resources to meet external demands. Mindfulness and emotional intelligence are inner resources that can help you deal with challenges and the stress of life." On the other hand, according to *Psychology Today*, a lack of resilience is associated with high stress, absenteeism, poor performance and mental conditions.[11]

What I found difficult to understand was the controversy around resilience – some believe that focusing on resilience somehow means accepting that negative conditions are okay because they are simply part of life, and this mindset ignores public responsibility. For example, some people who have experienced trauma get upset when resilience is brought up because they say that it puts the burden on the victims to simply accept that bad things happen in life and get over it, rather than placing the burden on the person who caused the bad thing to happen in the first place.

As Laura Bakosh puts it, "People think pushing resilience is victim blaming, yet they don't understand that developing resilience is life-affirming and helps one ride the waves of challenges and catastrophes." I see that as a good thing. Yes, the person who caused the trauma is to blame, but building resilience can help victims cope with their trauma, and that doesn't take anything away from public responsibility – they are not mutually exclusive. So, let's focus on what we do know, which is that people who have developed resilience are said to have an easier time coping and making decisions.

The American Psychological Association suggests "Ten Ways to Build Resilience," which include (among other methods):

- Having a positive self-concept
- Building confidence in one's strengths and abilities
- Taking decisive actions in adverse situations
- Keeping a long-term perspective
- Considering the stressful event in a broader context.[12]

JOURNALING BREAK:
Resilience

- What does perseverance mean to you?
- Write about a time when you were sad or angry, and then write about how you handled it. Did you handle it well? What could you have done differently?
- Think of a difficult challenge you went through recently. How did you overcome it? How did the experience help you to grow?

6

KINDNESS MATTERS

Living Together in Peace

Believing in yourself is a really good start in your journey to stressing less, but, of course, there's more to the story. In a time that is so chaotic, with people split on nearly every major issue and our world fracturing, how do we heal and attain peace? According to Andrew Jordan Nance of Mindful Arts San Francisco, "It takes a lot of work. Practice makes progress. We're never going to be perfect because we are works in progress. If we can just be kind when we have these big emotions, we can be more skillful with how we treat ourselves and other people. Keep cultivating kindness in yourselves, in your families, your friendships, and don't give into reactivity. Really cultivate wise action. You can either react blindly or respond wisely."

JUST SHOW UP

My Grandpa Jack put it simply when he said, "Smile, and the world will smile with you." (That has since become Wuf Shanti's kindness mantra.) In other words, smiling is catchy, and it's so easy to do. It's the start of so many kind gestures – making a new friend by reaching out, making an effort to be nicer and actually talking to each other more, helping someone when they need it, or helping the world somehow, like by volunteering with a charity. Any act of kindness, large or small, can create a ripple effect.

Community activist Shelly Tygielsky said that the "most important thing we can do in life is show up. That means in a whole way, even when no one else shows up or you don't feel like showing up. Don't get discouraged because if you keep showing up, you will make whatever your dream is come true. How we show up is also equally important, so commit to practicing every day. You will show up whole, instead of fractured, and what you are able to give out, you will get back." Shelly started meditating on the beach on Sunday mornings, and within a year, she had hundreds of people joining her. All she did was continue to show up, and from that, she developed a community comprised of people from all walks of life who respect and help each other. As Jessica Morey said, "Everyone has unique struggles, and we're not so different from each other, so knowing that, we can support each other. Respect each other." That's really all it takes.

But is it that simple? There has, of course, been a huge increase in violence to self and others, as well as a lot of bullying and isolation in the life of a teen these days. In the US alone, 1 in 4 teens reports being bullied; 9 out of 10 LGBTQ students experience harassment; 5 million students stay home out of fear of being bullied at school; almost 300,000 students are physically bullied in school each month; a third of students report having heard a classmate threaten to kill another student; and most teens believe that violence has increased on school campuses.[13] Anxiety, depression, anger and other mental health issues are the number one problem(s) reported by teens.[14] Where has the kindness gone?

People may not think that kindness is a big deal, but it can literally change the trajectory of the world. We can learn to be kind – to ourselves and others – and therefore reduce violence.

When I became a teenager, I was nervous about getting teased for Wuf Shanti, because I was playing this dog character. Wearing the costume made me self-conscious around my peers, and every time someone made a snarky comment, I wanted to say, "Well, we teach kids about how to be kind... so, do you want me to sign you up for a class?!" But responding with sarcasm would have escalated the situation, so I figured out a better way to deal with it. I did what Grandpa Jack taught me to do: I laughed. Remember, laughing – just like smiling – is catchy. They won't keep teasing if it doesn't seem to bother you.

CYBERBULLYING

The teasing I experienced does not come close to the amount or seriousness of the bullying that some kids have to deal with these days. Cyberbullying has really allowed such behavior to get out of hand because it does not stop once we leave school for the day; it's 24/7, in front of all your friends. Sports broadcaster and communication expert Dan Devone told me that the rise in severe bullying aligns with the timeline of when the smartphone was invented, and the best thing teens can do is unplug regularly, so they don't have to be connected to bullies at all times.

Phones and social media lead to detachment and loneliness, comparisons of your life to the seemingly perfect lives of others, and a willingness to be unkind. Psychiatrist and author Dr. Dan Siegel told me, "Social media is all about the 'me,' meaning the individual. We are meant to be in connection with each other and belong, not be isolated. The happy pictures on social media are an illusion. No one is happy like that. Other people think, 'OMG, I'm not like that,' and then they feel hopeless. We have to get people back in their bodies, back into their relationships with people and with nature."

Two tragic events, which occurred while I edited this book in 2022, hammer this point home: mass shootings at a grocery store and an elementary school, both of which caused an unimaginable loss of innocent lives. Both acts were carried out within ten days of each other by 18-year-old males, each of whom had used social media as a forum to discuss their plans. The isolation and rhetoric should have been an alarm to anyone who saw the posts, but because we have become so desensitized and "me-focused," no one reported them.

Everyone probably just scrolled past. We could have saved lives. We could have done – and can do – better. Social media is here to stay, so let's use it for good: Speak up and help others.

To learn to connect and love more, you can start by communicating with – believe it or not – the people who frustrate or annoy you the most. By sending love to those people, it will open your heart, make you to feel free and allow you to give even more love to yourself.

JOURNALING BREAK:
Social media

- What do you think about social media and the way it seems to depict picture-perfect lives?
- Do you think most people are showing their true selves and that everything we see on there is real?
  - Do you think other social media users are comparing their lives to other people's?
- How can you be more authentic with your posts?
- Do you believe that we have become desensitized to social media posts, that we scroll past red flags or that we do not report them because we don't want to be tattletales?

> ○ If so, how can you commit to doing better going forward? Can you say something if you see something?

Before the pandemic, I voluntarily got off all my personal social media accounts. Not only did I log off, but I also deleted the apps from my phone. I know it might be hard to believe, but I promise that my parents had nothing to do with this decision.

So... *why* did I do it?

Honestly, I felt addicted to my phone, like I always needed to look at it, and I spent too much time caring about what was happening on it. Being on it so much made me unhappy and negatively affected my mood. So, I ripped off the band-aid. It was hard at first because all my friends are on it, and that's how teens talk to each other these days, but it got easier. You only feel left out if you allow yourself to feel left out, or if you define yourself by social media.

I felt free, like I could breathe. I was happier, and I got time back – time to actually see my friends, face to face. (And if I couldn't see them in person, then I would call, text or FaceTime.) I also had time to ride my bike, play basketball and golf, and be with my family. The thing about phones is that they connect us more than ever before, but they actually disconnect us more than ever before, too. Believe it or not, I felt more connected to people when I was off my phone.

TAKE A BREAK

As Jennifer Miller of Confident Parents Confident Kids said, "We are alone with our phones and laptops. Our hearts sync up when we're eyeball to eyeball and connecting to one another. The less we're present with each other, the more disconnected we'll feel. That's one reason for the uptick in depression and anxiety. Consider unfollowing the consistent criticizers and judgers. Why do you need that toxic energy? It's not just you. Everybody, even the coolest person, feels scars from criticisms, so how can we be aware of that so that we don't add to those scars? Consider your own contributions. Are you criticizing, judging, adding fuel to the fire? Look at your own digital participation. Are you adding goodness to the world and your community, or are you bringing folks down and being part of the problem? We have to self-reflect as well."

When we make a choice to press pause on social media, there's no looking at people's perfect lives (which we all know aren't really perfect), and there's no unkindness to worry about (I didn't have much of that with my friends, but I know there are sadly lots of kids and teens that get cyberbullied).

It seems that teens – and most people, for that matter – really don't know how to communicate anymore. This generation is growing up with cellphones and social media, so looking each other in the eyes isn't a priority. Even when hanging out in the same room, we are all looking down at our phones. Now that I've experienced "looking up," I can definitely say that putting my phone down has helped me connect more with others.

JOURNALING BREAK:
Taking breaks and building connections

- Put your phone down for ten minutes, then come back to this prompt.
  - How did that break make you feel?
  - Can you commit to taking a ten-minute break daily?

- What happens when everyone starts talking at once? Can you hear what each person has to say? Can you focus on what your friends are telling you?
- How often do you truly listen to your friends when they talk? If you don't do so often, how can you improve this?
- Are you ever on your phone when simultaneously having conversations with people? How does it make you feel when someone is looking at their phone while you're talking to them?

My friend Janet feels pretty strongly about connecting with others and managing stress by speaking honestly and openly, especially when she has conflicts with friends. She explained that, in her junior year, she was under a lot of stress from school and breaking up with her boyfriend, and because her closest friends were hanging out with bad influences, which changed their personalities so much that she didn't want to hang out with them as much anymore. For a few months, she was really depressed.

So, Janet decided to disconnect from her phone for a while to focus on herself. She said that being on it so often was draining, but she had never shared her feelings openly with anyone before because of the pressure to be perfect and because she feared the judgment of others.

Turns out, Janet felt much better when she put down her phone and did something else. She had been so consumed with social media that she forgot to live her day-to-day life. And bottling up her feelings was worse than sharing them – she learned that by letting them out, her stress lessened. Through that, Janet also realized that stress is temporary.

Janet's recommendation to teens is to detach from the internet for at least two hours a day and go do something they truly love. When it came time for her to talk to her friends about the conflict they were having, she reached out and expressed her true feelings because getting those feelings out in the open – instead of keeping them inside – really helped her to feel better. One of the tricks she uses to live mindfully is asking herself if the problem (whatever is stressing her out) will matter in five years. If not, then it's probably not worth stressing over.

When I got away from social media, all the adults in my life said how proud they were of me, but more importantly, I was proud of myself. I stayed off those platforms for eight months, but I got back on when Covid happened so that I could keep in touch with friends. I'm admittedly on my phone a lot more, but I've still reduced my screen time because I'm more conscious of it. Again, I'm not telling you to delete everything because that would be super hypocritical of me, but like Janet, I am suggesting a balance.

Ways to cut down on screen time:

- Designate one day of the week to go offline – "phone-free Fridays," for example.
- Make a point to put your phone down for 15 minutes a day.
- Aim to have one face-to-face conversation each day.
- Connect in other authentic ways: take a walk; play basketball or golf or whatever your sport is; play chess or draw – whatever hobby you like to do with your friends; ask how another person is doing and really actively listen to the answer by asking follow-up questions.

Give it a few days, a week, and see what happens. You'll see you're not really missing out on anything; your close friends will understand and support you, and they'll still be there to talk to you about your day. You don't need social media to validate you or make you feel special and worthy, as long as you believe that you are special and worthy (which you are). It's up to us, our generation, to turn the tide toward more balance and real connection. Choose to believe in yourself instead of comparing yourself to the fake, picture-perfect lives we see on social media.

THINK BEFORE YOU POST

If you want to be successful or make positive change, then you also have to be conscious of what you post. Dan Devone talks about this point a lot and urges teens to "think before you post. Something can be dug up from years ago that you posted and haven't thought about since. It can change your life." Communication author Cory Alexander agrees. He said, "Everything teens do today affects tomorrow. What you do today really matters. When you're running for senator or want to be a principal of a school, and they do a background check… what you do today really affects you for tomorrow. Nothing ever goes away. Nothing ever deletes. Posting inappropriate pictures stays."

While I try to think of everything before I post, I'm human, like the next person, and I may make a mistake one day. Hopefully, whatever it is, it won't hurt anyone else or me. All I can do is try to commit to conscious posting and take a step back to pause before writing. I also acknowledge that it is impossible to make everyone happy all the time. There may be a group you didn't know about or a perception you didn't consider, and if that happens, I'd say to learn from it and resolve to be better. I don't ever want to be the cause of someone else's distress, and I'm sure you don't, either. Anti-bullying expert and psychologist

Dr. Laura Martocci said that "when someone is bullied, whether intentionally or unintentionally, shame lights up the same pain centers in their brain as does breaking an arm or any kind of physical energy."

WHAT TO DO WHEN YOU EXPERIENCE BULLYING

What should you do if you are being bullied, or when someone you know is being bullied? According to clinical social worker Patti Criswell, the first thing to do is to "never respond to the insult. Only respond to the act of being insulted." If you have been practicing mindfulness, then hopefully your self-esteem and self-confidence will allow you to hold tight to the knowledge that you are not what bullies say you are. We are all unique and special and deserving of love. Trauma psychologist Dr. Lee-Anne Gray shared with me a good mantra for times when we need strength: "Even though I am upset, and this is not okay, I can get through it."

Another important skill to learn, especially when seeing another person bullied, is to be an **upstander**. As anti-bullying expert Alexandra Penn explains, bystanders should be upstanders. "In every bullying equation, there's the bully, the bullied and the bystander. If someone speaks out on behalf of another – it only takes one person to start – then others will join in. There has to be an upstander in the group. Eighty-five percent of the time, if bystanders just stand up, it will stop." Teen advocate Elayna Hasty agrees. "You want to stand up for a bullying victim, be an upstander and tell the bully to stop. Invite the victim to walk away with you. Every seven minutes, a minor under 18 is being bullied, but only one-fourth of the time, someone intervenes. Kids and teens need to be more empowered to stand up for their peers and themselves."

It's not easy being an upstander – it takes a lot of courage. But you need to put yourself in that person's shoes, empathize with what that person is feeling, recognize how you would feel if you were the one getting bullied, and resolve to do the right thing and help. ABC News correspondent and *10% Happier* author Dan Harris taught me about a concept called "Wise Selfishness." He explained it simply, saying, "If you develop care for other people, you will be happier. If you want to have a better life, helping other people is the way to do it." Seems like being an upstander is a win-win.

JOURNALING BREAK:
Being an upstander

- What does the following phrase mean to you: "Do unto others as you would have them do unto you"?
- Write about a time you saw someone being mistreated for being different. How did it make you feel? What did you do about it – or what do you wish you had done?
- Do we always have to agree with others on everything we believe in? If not, how can we move forward while holding on to our values?
- What can you do when you hear or see someone else going through a difficult situation or getting bullied?
  - What if that person is not your friend, should you still help them?
  - What would you like for them to do if you were the one getting bullied?

I want to reiterate that I'm not blaming all the world's problems on cellphones or social media, and I fully recognize and appreciate that we need both to function in today's society. In fact, I'm grateful that I have a phone so that I can stay connected with my friends no matter what is happening in the world. All I'm advocating for is a balance. It's about mental health and kindness to ourselves and others. I'm sure I'll continue to take breaks from social media. My parents were thrilled, to say the least, that for eight months, I was not looking at the phone while I was talking to them or watching TV with the family. If we can be more aware of the world around us and reach out to help others, then we can spread kindness and stop the violence.

7

SURVIVE AND THRIVE

Putting Your Mental Health First

While I am a mental health education advocate, I am not professing to be an expert in all things mental health. As I write this, I'm 16… 17… 18… (a book takes a while from writing to editing to publishing), and I am not a psychologist. I haven't even started college yet (but will have by the time you are reading this). Also, the appropriate language and terminology changes often, so please forgive me if five years from now (or even tomorrow), there is a better way I could have or should have said something.

TRIPPING OVER WORDS

Language is really important, I know, but sometimes it can get confusing. For example, I once had a mental health expert tell me not to use the term mental *illness* and to say mental health *disorder* instead, and not even two hours later, when interviewing another mental health expert, that person told me not to use mental health disorder or illness and to say mental health *conditions* or *issues* instead. Both of these people are highly regarded, so it confused me as both the interviewer and as someone who is always trying to learn and understand what the right terms are. On top of that, the terms change with time too. So, as I said before, please know that everything comes with good intentions, and I hope you will agree that connecting with people and helping them is more important than the terms I use. To me, the main thing to understand is that we all deal with mental health, whether it's a diagnosable illness or not.

There are a lot of appreciation weeks or months to bring awareness to things, such as Mental Health Awareness Month, and that's great. We do also talk more openly about mental health than ever before. But we need to keep this conversation going every day to eradicate the stigma that's still attached to these conditions. As I said, everyone deals with mental health, so we need to make talking about it more of a regular, daily thing, and even make it part of school curriculum, so kids and teens know they are not alone.

A lot of people have hidden physical health problems that we can't see with our eyes, such as autoimmune conditions, and the same is true for mental health. If we all look to the right or left of us in school, we can be more or less assured the person in the next desk is dealing with something in their lives that we don't know about. I remember seeing a quote somewhere that I'll paraphrase because I don't know who said it, but it went something like, "People may act happy but not feel happy, act confident but feel nervous, look beautiful but feel less than." The point is that we don't know what anyone is going through, so we shouldn't judge, and we should always try to be kind.

ANXIETY AND DEPRESSION

It is essential that we treat our mental health just as we would our physical health and focus on keeping our minds and spirits healthy. Unfortunately, the number of teen suicides has risen dramatically in the past few years. Today's kids are dealing with depression, suicidal thoughts, substance abuse, trauma, trafficking, isolation, severe anxiety and more. Plus, teens are in between wanting to be treated like adults and still needing the guidance and direction from their parents and teachers. That's why, when it comes to mental health, it's imperative that we keep the lines of communication open. Mindfulness can help with that too.

JOURNALING BREAK:
How are you feeling?

- What are emotions? What emotions are you experiencing right now? Why?
- Do you notice when your feelings show on your face or in your body? Sometimes our feelings may show in our hands, feet or other areas. Where in your body do you notice your feelings?
- What happens to your body when you are stressed? How does your body feel when you are worried? How does your heart feel when you are sad? What happens to your focus, memory and decision-making skills?

The Centers for Disease Control and Prevention reports that one in five American minors ages 3 to 17 – about 15 million kids – experiences a mental, emotional or behavioral disorder in a given year. Only 20 percent of these minors are ever diagnosed and receive treatment; 80 percent, about 12 million, are not receiving treatment. Recent research indicates that serious depression is worsening in teens, which can lead to anger-management problems, violence and suicide.[15] In many teens, this depression – or other conditions, such as eating disorders – stems from their anxiety, and the average age at which it starts is getting younger and younger. There are plenty of resources: We can call helplines, write to get help from mindful organizations or read mental health books, but self-harm has still become a real threat, even for pre-teens. Because of this, more than ever before, we need to give students the tools to cope with emotions in a better way and let them know that they have a voice – and we hear it.

Worry, anxiety, stress and sadness are all natural and expected when it comes to mental health; so, the question is, at what point do these feelings become a problem? The truth is, the answer is different for everyone, and the answer can change in type and intensity at any point. You could be dealing with regular daily stress well, and then something could happen in your life that significantly challenges your ability to maintain your mental health. **If there's a sense of constant hopelessness or worthlessness, or if there's a pervasive lack of sleep or focus, that's a warning bell – reach out to someone for help.**

WHAT *EXACTLY* IS A MENTAL HEALTH ISSUE?

A mental illness/disorder/condition is when your life is being disrupted in a significant way, and it can be caused by lots of different things, including:

- Trauma
- Your environment
- Genetics
- Discrimination
- Abuse
- An injury
- A medical disorder...

... and more. It's important to know that mental health doesn't discriminate on the basis of age, religion, nationality, race, geography, socioeconomic status or anything else – it can affect anyone, anywhere, at any time.

Anxiety is when someone is unsure of themselves or a particular outcome. Everyone can relate to feeling anxious at certain times in their lives, such as when taking a test or starting a new school and having to make new friends. Unfortunately, chronic anxiety runs at a much deeper and more profound level for a large part of society. Chronic anxiety is more than just feeling anxious about an event – it's anxiety that can take over lives, and it's exhausting. For some, thriving through anxiety requires a lot of hard work, and that's why people are constantly looking for ways to better respond to it.

According to the Merriam-Webster dictionary, depression is marked by:

- Sadness
- Difficulty thinking or focusing
- An increase or decrease in sleeping and/or eating
- Feelings of being alone
- Hopelessness
- A lack of energy
- Sometimes, suicidal tendencies.[16]

There are an abundance of medications, therapies and techniques to manage depression, but we still need to teach mindful coping mechanisms to round out the care for this condition, since depression is such a prevalent problem.

MINDFULNESS MEETS ANXIETY AND DEPRESSION

When faced with anxiety or depression, mindfulness can be a helpful tool, and having a goal for the day of practicing for a few minutes can really help teens give themselves a break. Anxiety and depression are not flaws – we will likely experience some form of both at various points throughout our lives. For teens, we have to keep it real because, as I've said before, social media is filled with snapshots of what appear to be perfect lives, but the truth is that you never know what's going on with someone – and it's almost always different to what we see on the outside.

As Whitney Stewart points out, "Teenagers who practice [mindfulness] regularly will have decreased levels of stress and better methods of handling stress, less depression, more focus in school, and their grades improve. Think of it as changing your brain for the better." For some, depression and anxiety are daily battles, so practicing mindfulness routinely can help counteract negative thoughts and ground teens in the here and now, allowing them to focus on one day at time.

Emily Brierly, a teen who survived the 2017 bombing at Ariana Grande's Manchester concert, said that she was "in a constant state of fight or flight, and mindfulness meditation literally helped her become present." She made a conscious decision to practice so that she could find more moments of joy. Emily said mindfulness "completely stopped the panic attacks, stopped the anxiety, and that really helped her a lot."

My friend Lily was dealing with significant depression. She explains that the feeling hit her hard, and she felt like she was just going through life instead of living it. Her happiness depended on other people, so if they left, her joy did too. She realized she had to find happiness in herself and fight for herself – if her only reason for fighting was for someone else, then once they left, she'd have no purpose.

Journaling helped her a lot. She wrote down everything she wanted in life, and seeing her goals and dreams helped her realize what she wanted to live for. I'm not saying journaling cured her depression, but it helped her cope with it and find purpose.

What was also interesting to me is that Lily shared that she feels as if mental health in pre-teens is not taken seriously. For example, if people hear of a 10-year-old dealing with depression, they dismiss it by saying that someone that age is too young to be dealing with depression, so it must not be real or significant.

It's important to Lily that adults understand that mental health does not have an age limit and does not discriminate, so we need to support all humans, any time they open up to us. Rather than minimizing their emotions, listen and let them know that it's not only them, and it can be okay.

Just as Lily said, we are complex humans, and we are permitted to feel what we feel. Sometimes that may be more than one thing – both happy and sad, both joyful and fearful – and that's okay because we are not our emotions, just as we are not our illnesses. Scientists believe in the mind-body connection, which proves Grandpa's point that our thoughts have the ability to make us well or unwell, to lead us down a path of negativity or positivity. In fact, author Wayne Dyer backed that up when he said, "You cannot always control what goes on outside, but you can always control what goes on inside."[17] Mindfulness is a coping mechanism that can help us focus on one thing that makes us smile or lifts our spirits, and even if for only a moment, we are taking steps to train our brains. Pediatrician Dr. Dzung Vo believes that mindfulness can help every person, at every age, from kindergartners to high school seniors, with anxiety and depression. He said that "learning how to manage stress in a healthy and productive way will be a huge thing for our adult lives and will help us to be healthy and successful for the rest of our lives."

JOURNALING BREAK:
Letting go

- How do you release emotions so that you don't hold
  on to them and let them fester inside of you? Do
  you talk them out, write them out, dance, cry, sing,
  scream, use essential oils, play a sport, etc.?
- What do you think happens when we don't let our
  emotions out?
  - When we feel sad or angry, should we take it out
    on other people? Should we hurt ourselves or
    someone else? Why or why not?
- Sometimes, when we get upset, we say things we
  don't mean, or we do things that are not kind to
  ourselves or others. Do you think that's related to
  how we understand and accept our emotions? How?

TRAUMA

I know that mindfulness can help with anxiety and depression, for
sure, but a lot of people have questioned whether mindfulness
can help a teen – or anyone – who has experienced trauma.
Trauma affects the vagus nerve, which runs from the brain to the
abdomen and helps the nervous system stay balanced. That's why
unhealed trauma can cause emotional turmoil, like a rollercoaster.
By practicing mindful techniques to regulate stress, we slow our
heartbeats and feel calmer. Teens need space to feel what we
feel without judgment – that's how we will heal. First, we need to
recognize what we are feeling, and then we can work on healing it.

Curious about whether we can use mindfulness for that
healing, I spoke to psychologist Dr. Sam Himmelstein of the
Center for Adolescent Studies. I asked if there was a specific

way that we should be teaching mindfulness to a teen who has experienced trauma. He said, "If you know your student has been through trauma, you may not invite them to close their eyes. Or if you do, give them the option to keep their eyes open." This small change may help them feel more in control, and it's something I always try to remember to do when leading a mindful practice. Trauma survivors need to know that they have a voice, and that they are strong and courageous for getting through every day.

If you are dealing with loss or trauma, you are not alone. The Covid-19 pandemic caused this for a lot of people, and, as I write this, my South Florida community is dealing with a deadly building collapse in the nearby town of Surfside. In the face of these and other traumatic situations, Heather Stang, a grief counselor, teaches a really simple mindfulness technique called "showing yourself mercy. It's just bringing your hand to your heart. This can be if you're grieving yourself or if you're helping someone who is grieving." I found myself doing this in the days and months after my grandfather passed, and it seems so simple, but it really did help, maybe because it helped me feel more connected to him, or maybe because I was showing myself kindness.

There is no timeframe for working through a trauma. It takes everyone their own amount of time to heal, and that's another reason why we encourage daily practice.

Even some seemingly simple events, like the monthly code-red drills in school, which are intended to prepare students in the event of a shooting, can be traumatic because students are not told whether what's happening is a drill or real life. And after it's over, students are expected to go back to class and start taking a test, without so much as a mindful moment to collect their thoughts, come to a place of acceptance and calm themselves down. Lori Alhadeff of Make Our Schools Safe said that "we need to give students the tools and strategies to be able to deal with stress appropriately as they go through school. We need to be teaching students and teachers different techniques for them to be able to use after the code-red drill is over... to be able to go into a learning mindset."

In Florida, there is a rule that requires schools to teach five hours of mental health curriculum per academic year. Do I think that's enough? No, but it's a start, and it's better than zero. The mandate includes things like mindful practices, but also topics such as substance abuse and trafficking as well – more on that after a journaling break.

JOURNALING BREAK:
Handling trauma

Consider the following hypothetical, and how you would handle this situation:

You are about to sit down for a test and the code-red alarm goes off. You are not sure if it is a drill or for real. You evacuate the building. Your heart is racing, your breathing is shallow, you have a negative swirl of thoughts in your head. Thirty minutes later, everyone is allowed back into the school, and you have to sit down and take your test.

- What do you do? How do you get back into a clear and focused mindset to take your test?

ADDICTION

Here's the thing about teens: Even though we want to be adults, our brains are still not fully matured. The actual prefrontal cortex is still changing during adolescence, and that's the part of the brain that controls attention, impulse control and decision-making. Teens want immediate results and rewards, while adults are better able to take a pause and understand that not everything has to happen immediately. (I'm including myself in this, by the way.) How many times have you sent a text within 30 seconds of receiving one because you had to reply, perhaps out of emotion, and then you regretted what you sent? Or maybe you realized that you could have said it in a better way if there was a pause first? Or have you ever bought something you wanted in that moment, rather than saving up for something better because it would have taken you longer to earn more money? I remember seeing a post from Jack.org, a youth mental health organization in Canada, which said that teens are more likely to do homework to earn $10 immediately, rather than doing their homework in exchange for $100 that they'd receive a week later.[18] Our need for this instant gratification can get us into trouble, though.

After all, the late development of the prefrontal cortex is one potential reason why the statistics for self-harm and violence toward others is higher in our age group than in any other.[19] This means that an adult may stop themselves from doing something impulsive by thinking first about consequences, but a teen may not. Actually, some studies show that brain development can continue until we are in our 30s.[20] And that's a reason why the stats for addiction are so high too.

Steve Ronik, CEO of Henderson Behavioral Health, defines addiction as "when someone uses more of something than they intended to," and says that "early intervention is key. We know what to do about it and have great treatments for addiction now."

Usually, when people talk about drugs, they talk about things like cocaine, alcohol or opioids, but these days – and especially for teens – vaping is at the top of the list too. The Hanley Foundation's Diamond Howard says that "vaping is a drug; it does have high levels of nicotine, and is addictive. It can cause health issues like popcorn lung, seizures, and in some cases, death, and there is also the secondhand and thirdhand smoke that can affect the people around you in the community." When I spoke with teen Emanuelle Sippy about vaping, she said that "if vaping becomes our coping mechanism as teenagers, and we don't train ourselves to do something healthy as we get older, it will only bring worse coping mechanisms." She urges teens to "prioritize yourselves by eating well, staying hydrated and sleeping."

JOURNALING BREAK:
Healthy coping mechanisms

- Make a plan to deal with emotions. Write the following sentences in your journal, filling in the blanks with what works for you:
  - When I'm sad, anxious or upset, I will say _____ to myself (pick an affirmation)...
  - ... and I will go to _____ to find inner peace (pick a place that makes you feel calm and centered).
  - When I get to this place, I will take five deep breaths and think happy thoughts. I will return to my friends and family when I am feeling calmer and balanced.
- Make a plan to deal with situations that occur with friends if you believe they are in need of help, or that they plan to hurt themselves or someone else. Again, write the sentence below in your journal and fill in the blank to complete your plan.
  - When I hear my friend say anything that is a red flag or post anything that makes me concerned, I am going to tell _____.

I know it's going to sound weird, but vaping, alcohol and drugs are not the only addictions to consider. There's phone addiction, too – even the World Health Organization has recognized that teens are addicted to their phones and being online. Dan Devone agrees that there are new addictions such as video games, social media and, of course, our phones. He says, "Some teens today have no interest in sports, activities, friends or school anymore because they are addicted to being online. We need to find balance. Teens and young adults, 12 to 25 years old, are dealing with loneliness and detachment, and any time you're in that bubble, it becomes problematic, especially if we are constantly on our phones, because 95 percent of all communication is non-verbal, so if we are online excessively, it can lead to anxiety, depression and suicidal thoughts."

I know it may be hard to believe that phones cause us to be even more isolated and disconnected, or that there is a correlation with phone addiction, but the statistics don't lie. Steve Ronik opined, "It's important for young people to have a few others they can talk to and feel connected to. Something we can do at home to deal with stress is practice mindfulness." There are countless reports on mindfulness, and many of them show that this practice is most successful when it involves communication.

Marnie Grundman is a trafficking expert, and she said the number one thing she wants teens to know is to "talk to someone. The perpetrator is the person who should be ashamed, not you. One in five boys will be sexually abused by 18, and one in three or four girls. Ask yourself, 'Does anyone deserve that? Do I deserve that?' Abusers manipulate the victims into thinking they deserve it, but they don't. Everyone is going through similar insecurities, even adults. It only takes a moment to be kind, so take a moment every day and be kind to someone because that creates a ripple effect, and we'd have less problems in the world if we know it's okay to talk and listen to each other."

It seems like there is an underlying theme of communication, and that mindfulness is intrinsically tied to it. In fact, Diamond Howard's advice to teens about addiction is to "educate yourselves on the new trends because they change all the time, and they are dangerous, so know what's out there. Develop healthy coping mechanisms. Learn how to discuss feelings because if you can talk about it, you won't be as stressed, and [you'll be] less likely to turn to drugs. Really talk and listen to your friends because if you're really hearing them, you may save a life."

As part of the Mindful Kids Peace Summit, I interviewed more than 80 experts on different mental health-related topics, and I think the program was so well received because teens like to hear from their peers. I could have been saying the same thing as the adults in their lives, but somehow it makes more sense for them to hear it from someone their own age. Because I truly believe that teens are more likely to listen to their peers, I like to ask them what they think can help with mental health, addiction and self-harm.

A friend of mine, Johnny, began to feel sad constantly with very few glimpses of joy, and he used all his energy to mask it. He would put on a happy face for most of the school day, during extracurriculars and when he was with family, and then he'd be up at all hours of the night feeling hopeless and sad. It became worse and worse, eventually bleeding into his everyday life, as suicidal thoughts became almost constant.

He decided to talk to his parents about it, which was very difficult, and he began to see a psychologist. Johnny explains that the ability to talk to somebody about his feelings and have that outlet helped him a lot. Communication was essential for Johnny to effectively deal with his depression.

There are many traumatic experiences that teens may go through, and some may deal with addiction. All of that is very painful. Bob Roth, CEO of the David Lynch Foundation, told me, "We only use five to ten percent of the potential of the brain, and with stress, it's even less. In the toolbox of getting through life, [...] there should be an exercise to wake up your brain, to help steer through the trauma of the world. You don't have to feel overwhelmed. You can be happy."

The key things are to be present for others, talk to someone for yourself and know that it's okay to discuss mental health and emotions. Asking for help doesn't make us weak. I'd argue that it makes us strong and allows us to *thrive*.

8

FROM STIGMA TO FREEDOM

Out with the Old, In with the New

So, the consensus is that before we can learn how to manage stress and strong emotions, we first have to acknowledge that we have them, and that means talking about it.

DITCH THE SHAME

Traditionally, people have been afraid to talk about mental health, as if it's some kind of shameful secret. Mental health is nothing to be ashamed of – every single person on the planet deals with it at some point in their lives, whether they have general anxiety and depression or a more severe condition.

Thankfully, there has been a shift in recent years to eradicate the shame associated with mental health conditions. It is a welcome turn because people are starting to realize that **it's okay to ask for help.**

Think about it this way: If you broke your ankle, you would not be embarrassed to go to the emergency room for help. You should feel the same about asking for help with your emotions. Teen advocate Sophie Riegel said, "Shift your thinking from shame to how you'd like to feel, and say, 'I would like to feel calm,' and once you say that, you can start to manifest that feeling." This all starts by learning to talk about your mental health with acceptance and compassion and without judgment, which honestly may change the entire face of how you deal with your struggles, and how we actually end up lowering all the statistics – that, and true listening, because sometimes just listening can help someone, too.

Steve Ronik agrees. He said, "The most important thing is that people understand there's nothing to be embarrassed about. Mental health conditions among teens, and everyone, are super common, treatable, and people recover." He thinks it would be "really helpful if successful people talk about their mental health conditions because it's just a health condition like anything else. If someone had a heart condition, there would be no shame, they'd just talk about getting help for it. As more young people are comfortable talking about having a mental health condition, and what they did about it to get better, that's so powerful to other young people to hear that."

So, remember: **There is nothing to be ashamed of when it comes to your mental health.** The stigma of old is being replaced with compassion. Bottling up what you're feeling may lead to a tipping point. By talking about your experience, you may not only help yourself, but also help others who are dealing with similar issues or their own individual traumas. Hearing a story of survival from you may be just what they need to get through their own struggles.

When we say teens are not alone, we actually mean that in two ways:

1. It may not be the exact same experience, but everyone has experienced strong emotions, difficult issues, tough conditions and traumas, and there is more acceptance and compassion in the world than ever before. I know it may not seem like that sometimes, especially when you watch the daily news, but consider the fact that celebrities and

athletes are willing to share their stories and talk openly about mental health. That alone proves that you are not the only one in the world to have felt a certain way.

2. Studies have shown that you only need one person in your life to make you feel like you are not alone. According to Jennifer Miller, "Research says that in order for someone to be happier and have a sense of well-being, you only need ONE good friend." Find that person. It can be a friend, family member, guidance counselor or therapist. Take a minute to consider who that person would be for you – and then talk to them.

Todd Wolfenberg believes that "mental health is a very common thing that lots of people deal with on a day-to-day basis, even high-functioning, creative, successful people. Lots of people struggle with mental health, so it's not an isolated thing, and the more honest conversations we have, it will become normalized in society." And teen advocate Emanuelle Sippy agrees. She says that if "more people can start being open, honest and vulnerable, then we can create a cultural shift and overcome the mental health stigma."

ATHLETES CHANGING THE GAME

Many professional athletes are starting to speak up about their mental health. This is great because, just as I believe that teens will listen more to other teens, I also believe that when teens see their role models opening up and being vulnerable, they are more apt to listen. It gives us permission, in a sense – we know that it's okay to talk and there's nothing to be embarrassed about because even the best of the best struggle with ups and downs.

Here are just a few examples of athletes who have talked openly about or cared for their mental health:

- **Kevin Love**, a professional basketball player, opened up about his struggle with depression in 2018 when he wrote an open letter about it.
- **Naomi Osaka**, a tennis player, shared her history with severe anxiety and often skips press conferences to care for her mental health.
- **Simone Biles**, an Olympic gymnast, withdrew from some of the competitions during the 2021 Olympic Games to focus on her mental health. She said, "I say put mental health first because if you don't, then you're not going to enjoy your sport or succeed as much as you want to. We have to focus on ourselves because at the end of the day, we're human too, and we have to protect our minds and our bodies."[21]

We should applaud Simone and each of these athletes for their strength, courage and willingness to be vulnerable. This is really important because we will pay attention and listen to role models, and their openness will help end the stigma surrounding mental health issues. In sharing, they are helping so many other people.

Many professional sports players practice mindfulness themselves as part of their daily routines. In fact, many of them practice some form of yoga, meditation or mindfulness every day to help them deal with stress, focus, build endurance and stay healthy and grounded. They have coaches for strengthening and conditioning, nutrition and physical therapy, and many teams employ mental health coaches as well. Time is deliberately set aside each day to cultivate a mindful mindset and, if we consider how busy a pro athlete's training schedule is, we can see just how much they value this practice, and that we can choose to make time for it, too.

The Seattle Seahawks implemented a program called Mental Health Matters to let their players know that it's okay to not be okay, and it's okay to talk to someone about how they feel. They don't have to pretend that everything is perfect. NFL cornerback Sydney Jones IV is a big proponent of this program, and so is wide receiver Tyler Lockett, who wants people to know that it's okay to ask for help.[22] Super Bowl-winning quarterback Russell Wilson not only has a personal trainer, but also has a mental-conditioning coach who has him run through psychological exercises to train his mind.[23] In any sport – whether it is football for Russell Wilson or golf for me – the mental aspect of the game matters just as much as the physical. We need to develop skills for both, which that means working on our physical muscles and our mental muscles.

> **"I'm prepared, relaxed and ready. And this isn't just about basketball. It's about life. That's what mental fitness means to me."**
>
> **– LeBron James**

LeBron James has become a spokesperson for the Calm app because he is a strong advocate for mental fitness, and he has reportedly incorporated a mindful practice into his daily routine as well. So, just as he practices his game on the court daily, he also practices meditation for stress relief off the court. His mindfulness training strengthens the skill of focusing and helps him calibrate everything going on in his mind.

When asked what mental fitness means to him, LeBron said, "For starters, it means presence. No matter what I'm doing, my attention is locked. It means awareness. I can see my surroundings with clarity, and I can calculate my options. It means calm and composure, in those big moments when the pressure is on. It means resilience. I face a setback, and I show up fresh the next game. The next quarter. The next possession. It means I walk into a room, or step onto a court, and I'm at ease. I'm prepared, relaxed and ready. And this isn't just about basketball. It's about life. That's what mental fitness means to me."[24] This incredible athlete, who has won four NBA championships, understands that mental conditioning is key to his success – just as much as physical conditioning.

Another amazing athlete who practices mindfulness is pro golfer Jordan Speith, winner of the 2015 Masters Tournament. He takes time to work not only on his golf swing with his coach, but also on his mindset; specifically, he aims to be fully present on the course and have an attitude of gratitude. Speith practices visualizations of success and uses an imagery reel of where and how he wants the shots to go, thereby building his confidence.[25]

Some athletes have taken it a step further, such as Kevin Love, who started a non-profit organization that focuses on mental health. The goal of the Kevin Love Fund is to inspire people to live their healthiest lives and break the stigma around mental health. His organization started a national conversation and is currently working diligently to get mental health curriculum into schools.[26] According to Kevin, "Everyone is going through something that we can't see. Sharing what you're going through may be the most important thing you do. It was for me."[27]

WHAT WE CAN DO TO KEEP THE BALL ROLLING

I strongly encourage you, if you are feeling depressed, anxious or angry, to talk to a counselor, teacher or an adult you trust, and don't pretend you're fine when you aren't – that's just piling trauma on top of trauma. We text all the time, but the problem with that is that we don't talk to each other enough about how we are feeling. We need to share feelings with each other so we can process our emotions in a healthy way.

The reality is that we all have bad days, we all get anxious and sad, and we all feel stress and get overwhelmed. But if we are constantly thinking about our stress, then we can get stuck in that thought pattern. The key is learning to identify how we feel and cope with change and stress in a healthy way.

First, we have to understand that just as we are not our emotions and can have multiple emotions at the same time, we are also not defined by our mental health and can also be in two mental places at the same time. For example, what if someone is stressed about studying for the SAT, which is considered a standard stressor, but also has an eating disorder, which is considered a problem? Being stressed out for an exam is not an anxiety disorder, but having anorexia is considered a mental health disorder. We need to realize that a pair of mental states can – and often do – co-exist.

> Here's my own experience with this: I was studying for the SAT and completing college apps, which is stressful, but I was also going through serious grief after my grandpa passed away around the same time. At one point, I had to reach out to my guidance counselor and principal to let them know that I was exhausted from it all and ask for their help. They didn't think any less of me for it; instead, they helped me by listening and being supportive.

We also need to accept that we are not aliens floating through space all by ourselves. About 75 percent of people experience some form of mental health distress by the age of 25.[28] As I've said before, anxiety and depression are very common, and both are normal to experience. It's when these conditions start to affect daily life that we need to know that it's okay to open up and talk about it. But those aren't the only ways we can help ourselves through a mental health struggle.

Other methods for improving mental health:

- Eating better
- Resting more
- Surrounding yourself with people who bring out the best in you
- Staying away from drugs
- Exercising
- Doing activities you love
- Having patience with yourself
- Developing a regular mindful practice routine

HOW SCHOOLS CAN HELP

It's no secret that I think schools can – and should – teach us how to be mindful, and there are so many ways for them to do it.

Schools can offer courses in communications in which students talk to each other and practice sharing how they feel. This would help teens live more authentically – they'll know it's okay to be themselves because they have classmates who accept them for who they are.

It would also be smart for schools to implement a "coping with stress" curriculum. J.G. Larochette of the Mindful Life Project thinks mindfulness should be part of the daily school curriculum because "if we say that physical education is important and academic education is important, well, mental well-being education is the foundation of both of those, so mindfulness should be mandatory in schools." If we do this, then kids and teens can learn how to deal with their emotions in a better way, and if we practice these tools – use them as an automatic response to stress – then we will grow up to be happier and more mindful adults.

You might be thinking, "*Many schools have student-run clubs that meet after school and teach mindfulness.*" That's true… but it's not the same thing as it being part of the daily curriculum, accessible to all students. If math and science are required, then stress reduction, kindness, communication, social-emotional learning and conflict resolution should be too.

I spoke with Laurie Rich-Levinson, who was formerly on the Broward County School Board, and she shared with me that she thinks "we have to change the mindset of people" so they see "that mental health is as important as academic [success]." Broward County's former superintendent Robert Runcie created the "Superintendent's Mindfulness Initiative" in 2018, recognizing that, beyond academic achievement, "… the mental health and wellness of our students and staff are paramount, with mindfulness a key component for improving our lives."

JOURNALING BREAK:
Having the conversation

- How can we get more people communicating about mental health?
- Who do you talk to when you are feeling overwhelmed? Who can you reach out to for help? Make a list of those people.

HOW ADULTS CAN HELP

Imagine if you often felt like a cloud was over you, but you didn't know why, and you didn't know how to make the cloud disappear. This is the reality for so many kids with mental health issues who don't understand what they're feeling and why.

According to the American Academy of Child and Adolescent Psychiatry, children as young as preschoolers can show signs of anger and violent behavior, and parents should not dismiss it as a phase that will end; instead, they should pay attention to their children and work on preventing that behavior from becoming commonplace.[29] The same goes for parents and educators of older kids and teens – they can help us cope, whether that's through making sure we know it's okay to talk about our problems; by being a supportive person we can talk to who won't judge us; or by practicing mindfulness. Dan Harris advises parents and teachers, "If you're interested in having mindful teens, you have to model it." Be the person that you want your son or daughter to grow up to be. He also shares that he did "nothing that his parents told him to do, but he does everything that they modeled," and he thinks "the most powerful thing you can do for your teens on this front is to model mindfulness. Your teens will pick up on it, and you'll be happier."

I think this applies to all role models, including educators. Think about it: If teens are learning mindfulness, but then they go into a classroom, and the teacher is stressed out and yelling, then how can the teens stay in a mindful headspace? It's a cycle, so it's essential for all of us to practice these techniques – we all influence each other, whether we realize it or not. Teen Sophie Riegel talked to me about the old saying, "Put your own mask on first," (and she said that before masks became a Covid thing), and it's so accurate, especially for parents or teachers or role models or activists who are using their voices to better our world. Simply put, we can't presume to help others if we don't take care of ourselves first.

> **"Parents and teachers, what you need to do is just be there to support us. It's not your job to fix us. We don't need fixing. We just need support."**
>
> **– Sophie Riegel**

Sophie went on to say, "One way to prevent mental health conditions is to get help before you need it. Everyone, no matter who they are, should be speaking to someone. You want to have a system in place when you are feeling good, so you know what to do when you're feeling bad. For teens, know that there are millions of others like you who are dealing with the same thing, so you aren't alone, even when it may feel like you are. For parents and teachers, what you need to do is just be there to support us. It's not your job to fix us. We don't need fixing. We just need support."

When I travel to schools and hospitals, I meet a lot of great people. Once, a sophomore – let's call her Abby – came up to me after a presentation I gave and thanked me. She said that she was a suicide survivor and that mindfulness brought her back from the edge, effectively saving her life. Abby told me that part of what helped her was being able to talk about her problems and feeling like she had someone who supported her in learning these techniques. Knowing I was able to make an impact on one person left a significant imprint on me, and I'm grateful that she shared her experience with me. And, though I'm sure Abby's not happy all the time – which is totally okay – I'm so proud of her for finding balance and calm in the midst of the storm.

A MORE MINDFUL GENERATION

It's true that focusing on what matters to you, finding what helps you feel balanced and implementing self-care can truly change your life for the better. Psychologist and Harvard Medical School professor Dr. Chris Willard had an uplifting prediction when we spoke. He said that learning mindfulness to calm ourselves makes us stronger against whatever stresses come our way, and if we can learn this stuff when we are young, then we'll save ourselves from a lifetime of pain and challenges. He said, "We're going to see a generation that doesn't end up with anxiety [and] depression at the same level, and see less violence, and we're going to see a more compassionate, more mindful, much healthier generation."

I hope he's right, but I do understand that teenagers have so much going on in our lives that we can become overwhelmed. We wish to grow up so that we can be independent, but that may be a case of "be careful what you wish for," because even though we will have more control over our lives, as adults, we will also have more responsibilities. So, we need to learn how to deal with pressures now, how to juggle different roles, and how to handle emotions in the face of obstacles so that we're really ready to grow up because, spoiler alert, all of these skills will only become more useful when we're adults.

So, where do we start? Matt Dewar of Journey 30K told me that "the first step for teens to reclaim their well-being is to slow down. Teens live at a pace that's not sustainable. Parents, teachers and coaches need to slow down too. Young adults need to focus on prioritizing. Students think everything is urgent. You can't live that way. What's actually important and worth your time?"

Good question. I actually think about this a lot. With schoolwork, test prep, being on the golf team, serving as president of the mindfulness club, speaking and teaching for Wuf Shanti, writing this book, having two jobs, spending time with family and friends, and finishing all the extra projects that people ask me to do, I have a lot going on, and sometimes I feel overwhelmed and have to remind myself that I can't do everything at once.

When I think about Matt Dewar's question – what's worth our time, which is our most valuable resource – I have to think about my purpose, because it is intrinsically connected. Right now, my purpose is helping others by teaching them different ways they can deal with stress and cope with emotions. It's vital to me that I make a difference.

Something happened after the TEDx Talk I gave. During intermission – right after I gave my talk – I walked out into the lobby, and a young girl, about seven years old, ran up and hugged me. Her mom explained that her husband, the girl's dad, was dealing with bipolar disorder, and that it'd been hard for them, but that my talk had helped the little girl understand what was happening to her dad. Having to deal with such heavy stuff at home is not easy, but I'm hopeful that she at least walked away with some helpful hints for processing her emotions and stress in a healthy way. I don't know what happened to her father, and I really hope he ended up being okay. I also hope that the little girl grows up to practice some daily mindfulness to help her cope with everything.

So, as I said at the start of this chapter, by ditching the shame associated with mental health, we gain control, balance and a community. Talking about it – and seeing others be open – helps everyone. It's imperative that all of us take care of ourselves by communicating our feelings so that we can be healthier and happier – more on that in the next chapter.

9

CARING ABOUT SELF-CARE

How Physical Health Affects Mental Health

We can't forget to take care of our bodies as we focus on our minds and spirits, which is often a hurdle that teens, myself included, need to accept and overcome. Gina Biegel of Stressed Teens urges us to remember to implement regular self-care techniques. "It's not selfish to take care of yourself. You can't care for anyone else if you don't care for yourself. We need to rigorously take care of ourselves, so we don't burn out."

You also need to remember to send yourself some gratitude every day because life isn't always easy, and part of self-care is treating yourself with the same love and compassion that you would give to another person who is suffering or struggling to thrive. So, check in with yourself and take inventory on how you feel, ask yourself what you need in terms of support, reach out and ask for help, and applaud yourself when you post about having a bad day, knowing that it's okay to live your life authentically.

PHYSICAL HEALTH

While our minds can control our bodies, we are also responsible for eating healthily, getting enough exercise (whether through team or individual sports), and getting enough sleep.

In fact, Dr. Diane Gehart told me, "If we don't have five things in place, it's going to be hard to have stable long-term happiness:

- Sleep
- Eating healthily
- Exercise
- Stress management, and
- Safe relationships.

The human body does much better when you're eating whole, unprocessed foods. Refined sugars and chemicals really affect the brain in a negative way, and that affects moods and causes anxiety or depression. So, we have to be mindful of what we are putting into our bodies and make sure to eat healthy. And we are a sleep-deprived society. Your brain is growing until you are 25 or 30 years old, and it needs at least nine or ten hours of sleep in middle and high school. The magical time to go to bed is 10:30pm. If you stay up later, then you'll be up until 2am because of the adrenaline. We also need 30 to 60 minutes of exercise five or six days per week. It boosts brain growth. It helps to prevent anxiety and depression and makes us feel better."

Um… I consider myself a mindful teen, but I definitely do not eat extremely healthily (my diet consists mainly of chocolate chip cookies), nor do I go to bed by 10:30pm (more like 12am), and I don't exercise for an hour six times per week (unless you count golf, but even that is maybe twice a week).

I guess we all have a lot more that we can be doing for our health. Scientists and doctors have said in numerous studies that exercise helps us to release anger and cope with emotions. It's essential that we recognize and appreciate the mind-body-spirit connection by eating, exercising and sleeping mindfully, and that we know there are plenty of ways to practice mindfulness that do not include traditional meditation. For example, when I go to the golf range, I practice my golf swing and focus only on being there in that moment, and that is a form of mindfulness because it helps me center myself and relax. Turns out, any activity that requires this type of concentration – and it doesn't just have to be yoga or meditation – can create positive mental health benefits.

Reduce stress:

- Take a break. Breathe.
- Move. Get outdoors.
- Nourish yourself. Eat healthily.
- Relax. Make time to unwind. Listen to music.
- Stay in touch. Connect with others.
- Ask for help. You are loved.

Take care of your body:

- Get enough sleep – at least 8–10 hours.
- Exercise. At least three times a week. Sports count.
- Maintain a balanced diet. Add in some healthy foods.
- Avoid tobacco, alcohol, vaping and drugs. Say no.
- Limit screen time. Look up.
- Relax and recharge. Even a few minutes every day of yoga, meditation, breathwork, mindfulness or affirmations will help.

Build support and strengthen relationships:

- Make connections. Join a support group.
- Do something for others. It will come back to you.
- Support a family member or friend. Make a positive difference in someone's life.

A good friend of mine, Bob, was feeling a lot of stress because of school, and he started working out – running every day – and going to bed at an earlier hour. Now, he says that he feels a lot better about everything, and these are some of the things that have helped him cope. If he stops doing them, then he starts to feel stressed again, so he sticks with this self-care routine.

Just like Bob, radio personality Joe Lockett says that he "works out to deal with stress, goes to bed early and leaves the day behind." He encourages teens to "say, 'Okay, I did all I could today, I gave my all, and I'll deal with the rest tomorrow.'"

Many studies have shown the positive effects that the proper amount of sleep, a healthy diet, meditation, yoga, exercise and positive thinking can have on the body and mind. With all of these proven benefits, why isn't everyone meditating, doing yoga, and eating, sleeping and thinking well?

Amy Burke of MindWell Education has an answer. She said, "Sometimes, our thinking mind can trip us up a little bit. If you're overthinking or worrying about something, you can get caught up in it. Like if you text someone, and they don't text you back, your thinking mind can be helpful but also unhelpful [...] if it's in the past or future. But our body is in the present moment, and so something like tapping or another mindful physical practice can help us to bring our brains back to now." Here are a few other ways to re-center yourself in the present.

HUMMING

When humans are stressed out, we tend to get sick more often, sleep too much or too little, and experience stomach discomfort, chest pain or other physical imbalances. For example, when we're stressed, our breathing tubes can spasm, so our bodies make nitric oxide in the paranasal sinuses, and that helps expand the breathing tubes to help with inflammation in the body and fight off diseases.[30] There is an activity that you can do to increase nitric oxide and ward off that inflammation... humming. Yup, I know it sounds funny, but you can hum to help your physical body – for example, when you have a sinus infection and want to breathe better – and to slow down your nervous system and help calm your mind. We hum all the time anyway, like when we sing, for example, so why not try it with intention?

HUMMING PRACTICE:
Mindful humming

- Inhale through your nose and hum on the exhale. I like to imagine the smell of the ocean air, but you can think of any of your favorite scents. One person told me that she likes to imagine the smell of the hair salon, and another person enjoys her grandma's banana bread. Use whatever works for you.
- The hum on the exhale should be natural, meaning not too high or too low in pitch.
- Do this a couple of times a day and see how it makes you feel.
- Do you feel calmer afterward? How about those sinuses?

THE EMOTION CODE

Something called the Emotion Code has also captured my attention – and yes, it fits in this chapter about physical health. That's because the Emotion Code gives you the ability to release your emotions to help with physical ailments as well.

After I met with Dr. Bradley Nelson of Discover Healing, and he performed the Emotion Code on me, I became a believer – so much so that I decided to get certified in the Emotion Code. I believe this is a very healing technique, and it allows you to feel lighter, better and like you're in a more positive space. It truly is awesome to witness!

The Emotion Code is based on the theory that the mind – possibly our subconscious mind, too – may really affect the body. As an Emotion Code practitioner, I believe that emotions can get trapped inside of us and potentially cause physical or mental conditions. It's like emotional energy that sits and festers in the body until it is released. The emotions come from a specific time or event that was experienced, either by you or someone else from whom you inherited or absorbed the energy. It may be from something that happened when you were three years old, or even energy passed down from an ancestor. The premise is that all these emotions can be released and may help you to feel better, and the Emotion Code teaches you how to let them go.

I tried the Emotion Code to help my friend's dad with his shoulder, which had been hurting for a few weeks, and he said that the pain actually went away afterward. I've experienced this myself, too, when I was having knee pain while also feeling a lot of stress and anxiety for seemingly no reason. After doing the Emotion Code and releasing those pent-up feelings, I felt lighter – like my true self.

It's not healthy to hold in our stress, and the Emotion Code theorizes that not only is it okay to release our emotions, but it's necessary in order to overcome the overwhelm. Dr. Bradley Nelson said that "the heart is like a brain and can remember and feel, and about 90 percent of physical pain people have is because of their emotional baggage. So, if you release the trapped emotions, you can heal physically and mentally."

JOURNALING BREAK:
Checking in with yourself

- What do you do to keep your body healthy?
- What are some of the things that make you happy?
- What activities can you do to help center yourself and find a sense of calm?
- What are some nice things that you'd like others to do for you when you're feeling stressed? And what are some things that you could do to support yourself and help yourself feel better?

HEART AND BRAIN –
ONE AND THE SAME

Jenna Moniz, an educator in Broward County, agrees with Dr. Nelson that the heart is actually like a second brain, as it has a memory and makes decisions. She said that while "many of us rule by our brains, we should make decisions of the heart because there is an intelligence of the heart, and it's 5,000 times more powerful electromagnetically than the brain, so if we shift focus to the heart, then we'd find more intuition, more compassion and more empathy." Jenna believes that "if we are constantly in fight-or-flight mode, then it wreaks havoc on the body, so we need to express our emotions. If you have bottled-up feelings and emotions that you're not addressing or expressing, they will do harm." She explains to her students that they can "express emotions in many healthy ways, whether that's writing about them, talking about them, going to the beach, crying about them, dancing, singing about them – as long as it gets the flow of energy going. It's all about energy."

I don't know if Jenna even knows about the Emotion Code or realizes that she follows the theory, but I've noticed that a lot of mindfulness practitioners believe in the heart-brain energy concept to release emotions, even if they don't use the words "Emotion Code." For example, when I was speaking with J.G. Larochette, he said that "when someone doesn't feel good on the inside, they are going to look for ways to make them feel better on the outside, like drugs, alcohol [or] social media, which are all unhealthy coping mechanisms. But if we teach teens how to recognize, accept and process emotions in healthy ways, it will allow for them to be authentic. Your authentic self is your real self, and that's what we want to see, so you don't have to act or be any different. If you are depressed or anxious, it's okay to feel it because it's part of our human beingness. Emotions are to be felt, not avoided. If we can process them in healthy ways, then we can release them and move beyond them."

LISTEN TO YOUR BODY

Just as our physical health can help with our mental health, so too can our mental health help with our physical health. We have to be cognizant of the fact that they are intricately connected.

I've always said that I'm a normal teen, even when people note how mindful I am. Yes, I know how to control my stress, but sometimes it's hard even for me.

The year 2020 was a rough one. My grandpa died from cancer, we were stuck in the house because of the Covid-19 pandemic, my great-grandma died from Covid-19, and, of course, I still had all the old stressors of homework, grades, work, extracurricular activities, relationships, the SAT, college applications and working on Wuf Shanti. Plus, I was in the midst of an evidenced-based study on the Wuf Shanti curriculum, I was writing this mindfulness book for teens, and I was recording audio meditations and videos for Inner Explorer and Stressed Teens.

It was a lot, I know, but I didn't really think I was stressed. I mean, I didn't feel stressed, or maybe I wasn't aware that I was stressed. It's funny because I'm a mental health advocate, and it turns out that I was unknowingly experiencing huge levels of anxiety.

So, how did I figure it out?

When I went to get the first Covid vaccine shot, I felt totally fine – not stressed or nervous at all… BUT my blood pressure was so sky high that they told me it was almost stroke level! *"What?!"* I laughed. Honestly, I thought their machines were broken, even though they took my blood pressure four times, and it repeatedly said the same thing. The nurse kept asking me if I was nervous, and I kept saying that I wasn't, which was totally true… in my mind, anyway. My body was telling me another story. My subconscious mind was obviously very anxious. After I got the vaccine shot, they took my vitals an hour later, and my blood pressure was normal once again.

This was the moment I realized that maybe I wasn't as self-aware as I thought: *"If I don't even know when I'm stressed, then how can I control it?"*

Thousands of scientific studies have been done showing the benefits of mindfulness, and many of them focus on physical effects, such as, ironically enough, lowering blood pressure. So, we know mindfulness helps with physical symptoms. But, as we know from the SEL studies, self-awareness is an important precursor, because if I didn't know that I was stressed to the point of potentially having a stroke, then I wouldn't know to do a mindfulness practice that would have been able to calm me.

Now, contrast that experience with the first time I ever took the SAT, which just so happened to be the week after my Covid vaccine. Wow, did I *feel* stressed! I KNEW that I was feeling super anxious. (As an aside, I'd really like to make a case to the College Board about getting rid of the SAT because I don't think standardized tests really measure anything, and they only stress and overwhelm teens at a time when they already have enough going on in their lives, but that may be an argument for my next book.) My mom decided to take my blood pressure with a cuff we had at home, expecting the same high levels from the week before when I was getting the vaccine. I was shocked that the blood pressure reading was normal! I took it a second time because, once again, I thought the machine was broken, albeit in the opposite way! And again, I got a normal result. All three times.

What did these experiences teach me? That when I feel stressed, my blood pressure is fine, and when I don't feel stressed, my blood pressure is sky high? Not *quite*. Instead, I realized that I have to do a better job working on my self-awareness and figuring out what my subconscious is up to, and that my body – just like yours and everyone else's – can give me clues if I learn to listen. But here's the biggest lesson I learned: Maybe I have to remember to practice what I preach, meaning, like, on a daily basis!

Sometimes, I get so busy that I forget my mindfulness practice for the day, and sometimes, if I'm feeling great, then I won't feel the need to do a mindful practice. At the same time, I tell everyone else that they should try practicing for at least five minutes every day. I used to do it, so why did I stop? Did I think I was immune to the effects of stress? Well, apparently, I am not. And did I think that I was adept at always recognizing my stress levels? Yup, I did.

I guess this was a good lesson at the time – and a good reminder for me as I write this book. Last night, before I went to sleep around midnight, I asked my mom to sit down with me and do a gratitude practice, a heartfulness practice and a chakra practice (which you'll learn more about in Chapter 10). It literally took us ten minutes from start to finish, maybe less, to be thankful, surround ourselves in light and send kindness to ourselves and others.

I was also reminded of how crucial it is to do our own practice(s) when I sent out a newsletter to my Board of Advisors for Wuf Shanti, who are mentors and guides, and many of whom are in the same industry as I am. I was grateful to see how many people wrote me back and said the same thing: They all go through bouts of anxiety and stress, and **it's normal.**

Yes, we understand the importance of self-care, but everyone – including mental health practitioners and advocates – needs to remember to make mental (and physical) health a priority and send ourselves compassion. We have to take time for ourselves to relax, be in a calm headspace and practice what we preach so that we don't burn out and can continue being leaders and helping others.

For me, right now, I think this means going back to the five-minute rule, even when I'm busy or feeling totally fine. Starting now. Again. Every moment is a new opportunity to start over. One of the core tenets of mindfulness is simply beginning again. And even the most mindful of us have to take a deep breath and begin again sometimes. I'm filled with gratitude that I have that opportunity.

PART 2

HOW CAN WE STRESS LESS?

10

MINDFUL TECHNIQUES

Coping with Stress and Emotions

So, now we know why we need to stress less, but how do we start *doing* it? How do we get to a more mindful place and deal with our feelings?

> **"The power you have is your brain."**
> **– Dr. Rick Hanson**

First, let's get one thing straight: Some people may think that by practicing mindfulness, we're trying to stop all thoughts, but we're not. Gina Biegel explains that we are going to always have random, sometimes negative, thoughts, but "it's more about what you do when you notice those thoughts because we can make our problems a lot worse by hanging on to them." So, you can choose to let a negative thought take up space in your brain and ruminate on it for hours, but that would be really unproductive and wouldn't accomplish anything except making you feel bad. The trick is not to allow what happened before or what hasn't happened yet to gobble you up inside. Mindfulness is like a superpower. Dr. Rick Hanson says, "The power you have is your brain. No one can stop you from what you focus your attention on and how you relate to it, and no one can do it for you."

JOURNALING BREAK:
Examining your thoughts

- How often would you say that your mind thinks of something negative?
  - How does consciously changing those thoughts make you feel each time?
- Set a timer for two minutes. During this time, write down every thought that pops into your head.
  - How many of the thoughts were about things you can control?
  - How many were about things that have happened in the past?
  - How many were about things that could happen in the future?

"The mind wanders. Get used to it."

– Dave Smith

A lot of people get frustrated in the beginning because they keep getting distracted by thoughts that jump into their brains when they are practicing. I asked Dave Smith about that once. He said, "The mind wanders, get used to it." He went on to say that "mindfulness is not about clearing the mind; it's about changing the relationship that we have with our minds. We do this because we want our minds to be friendly companions. The whole game is recognizing that our minds wander, and then bringing them back to the present moment. That's what mindfulness is all about."

In other words, you have all the control in this situation. With practice and acceptance – and without judgment – you get to control your thoughts, and that, in turn, helps you control your emotions and get your stress in check.

MINDFULNESS-BASED STRESS REDUCTION (MBSR)

Mindfulness-based stress reduction (MBSR) is a great tool to learn when you're young, so you can hone the techniques and use them whenever you need them later on in life. Considering that the average person has 50,000 random thoughts each day,[31] some of them are bound to be negative, and sometimes it's hard to stop the negative loop in your head. We simply have to learn how to watch them float by without attachment or judgment. Remember: The trick is to simply **begin again.**

There are so many different kinds of mindful practices that you can choose from, and it is important for me to reiterate here that these techniques can be done in just a few minutes, all without anyone ever knowing you're doing them.

Different techniques work for different people. Mindful art, or focusing on a creative art project, is a good practice, as are self-reflection prompts. If you like music, you can practice by putting on a song and focusing on a specific sound, like the drum beat or guitar riff. Personally, I like to listen to music while I'm golfing, a sport that already requires great focus. Adding music to that makes it like meditation – it helps me find peace, which then spreads to my parents, teachers and friends.

Try any of the following techniques, find which ones you like, and make them part of your daily routine. They will help you be better prepared to face all the ups and downs of life.

BREATHWORK

Inhale and exhale slowly.

If thoughts come, it's okay; the trick is to let them go and come back to the breath.

Your breath can be your anchor.

Breathing is good because it's calming – taking **slow, deep breaths** has the potential to prolong our life by years. Kevin Hawkins of MindWell Education believes that "we all move too fast. It's such a fast world. We spend a lot of time in our heads. All this energy in the brain, sometimes we just need to pull it down in the body and slow down. We know from neuroscience that these kinds of activities give us the ability to activate the part of the body that slows us down and take a breath. We can use the senses and the body to ground ourselves in the present moment."

Here are three ways to practice with breath:

BREATHWORK PRACTICE:
Count and hold

Something as simple as a deep breath in for a count of four, holding it for a count of four, and then releasing it for a count of four can help us feel calmer. We can do this while focusing on a beautiful light in a color of your choice and/or a positive thought.

- Pro tip: Try this deep-breathing technique before a test to help yourself focus and relax, and no one will even know you're doing it.

BREATHWORK PRACTICE:
Clean air

A second way is to visualize yourself breathing in clean oxygen and releasing stale carbon dioxide on the exhale.

BREATHWORK PRACTICE:
Breathe in peace – and breathe out to share it

The third way is to imagine that, when you're inhaling, you breathe in love and peace, and when exhaling, you're releasing all your worries.

Similarly, a technique I like is to breathe in love and peace for yourself, and then breathe out love and peace to the universe.

Choose whichever of these calls to you and give it a try. Or you can put them all together in one practice, like this:

BREATHWORK PRACTICE:
De-stress with your breath

- Close your eyes if you feel comfortable doing that, or gaze downward at the floor.

- Slowly breathe in, hold, and then breathe out, each for a count of four:
  - In: 1... 2... 3... 4...
  - Hold: 1... 2... 3... 4...
  - Out: 1... 2... 3... 4...
- Next, breathe in, envisioning beautiful, clean oxygen filling up your body; hold; then breathe out, imagining that you're exhaling all the stale carbon monoxide:
  - In: 1... 2... 3... 4...
  - Hold: 1... 2... 3... 4...
  - Out: 1... 2... 3... 4...
- Next, breathe in peace, love and kindness; hold; then breathe out, releasing all your worries and negativity:
  - In: 1... 2... 3... 4...
  - Hold: 1... 2... 3... 4...
  - Out: 1... 2... 3... 4...
- Again, breathe in peace, love and kindness; hold; then breathe out peace, love and kindness to the universe:
  - In: 1... 2... 3... 4...
  - Hold: 1... 2... 3... 4...
  - Out: 1... 2... 3... 4...

Knowing that today is a great day, and everything is okay... feeling grateful for the time you took for this practice... take a deep breath, then release it, opening your eyes when you're ready.

How do you feel?

Parent coach Sue DeCaro of Conscious Parent Thriving Kids says that the "quickest method to live a mindful life is [to use] your breath. These are lifelong skills that we are developing...

I can't think of anything more powerful in life than learning how to regulate our own emotions and control our own feelings and thoughts."

MINDFUL MUSIC

Mindful music is taking a moment to truly sit with the music, experience how the sound makes you feel, and be present with the lyrics or the beat as they resonate through your body.

MINDFUL MUSIC PRACTICE:
Your song

Simply listen to your favorite song at least once per day. That's it. Easy.

Choose a song that's uplifting and makes you feel good. Pick one sound to focus on, like the drumbeat or the guitar. You can also pay close attention to the lyrics. For example, Jason Mraz has a song called "Living in the Moment" with lyrics that help me remember to be present.

You can make your song practice even stronger by incorporating some breathwork at the same time. Remember to breathe in and out love and peace.

And remember that it's okay if thoughts come and go. You can acknowledge them and then release them without judgment, bringing your mind back to the present moment and the song – and begin again.

If on day one of your song practice, you have 500 random thoughts intrude, then on day two, you have 499, don't be discouraged – **that's still progress**. In fact, it's great, and you should be proud of that. The more you practice, the better at it you'll get it. And the next time a situation gets stressful or you're coping with some overwhelming emotion, you can listen to that song and be in the present moment with it, taking your mind out of the past or future, centering yourself in the present and getting to neutral, which allows you to be in a mentally happier place.

MINDFUL ART

Just like music, art is a great mindful practice. Find things that make you happy and things that relax you. That way, when you do these things, you're living in the moment and focusing on your activity, rather than the other noise in your head.

Coloring is actually a mindful meditative activity that can help people of all ages feel a sense of inner calm. You can amplify these effects by coloring symmetrically circular designs called mandalas, which help focus your attention, therefore teaching mindfulness and relieving stress and anxiety. According to the Mandala Project's website, mandalas "represent wholeness, and can be seen as a model for the organizational structure of life itself – a cosmic diagram that reminds us of our relation to the infinite, the world that extends beyond and within our bodies and minds."[32]

Mandalas can be found everywhere in nature and around us, even in flowers, sunshine and snowflakes. People of all ages can spend some time drawing or coloring mandalas, in quiet or with some soft music on in the background. There are adult coloring books with mandalas of all different shapes, some with animals or positive affirmations. While we're coloring, our breath regulates, and our brains are focused on the activity with a clear mind. We tune into the present moment.

JOURNALING BREAK:
Color choices

- Write down the thoughts or emotions come up when you focus on the following colors:
  - Red
  - Blue
  - Purple
  - Yellow
  - Green
  - Pink
  - Turquoise
  - Lavender
  - Black
  - Teal
  - Brown
  - Orange
  - White
- Is there a specific color that you gravitate toward? Why? How does it make you feel?

Recall once again how the mental and physical are connected. You drink water to keep your body healthy, right? The next practice comes from Stressed Teens, and it will require you to imagine your mind as a water bottle – and how you can fill it with things that keep your mind healthy.

MINDFUL ART PRACTICE:
Drawing your water bottle

- Draw a water bottle – make it large enough to cover your entire sheet of paper.
- Next, fill it with things that make you happy. You can draw them, or simply write the words.

When you're feeling sad or upset, you can look at that water bottle as a reminder to:
- Focus on those positive aspects of your life
- Take care of yourself by enjoying one of the things you drew in the bottle.

Drawing and coloring can also be combined with other mindful practices, such as our next technique, affirmations and mantras.

POSITIVE AFFIRMATIONS AND MANTRAS

We all have the ability to choose our thoughts. Choosing positive thoughts:

- Challenges our natural negativity
- Boosts our self-confidence
- Reduces our anxiety
- Helps us cope with emotions.

Some people like to write down their positive thoughts as statements and repeat them out loud as **affirmations**. If you practice this often enough, you will start to believe your affirmations, and they become true to you.

AFFIRMATIONS PRACTICE:
"I am"

Try an "I am" practice, meaning that your affirmations will all start with the phrase "I am." For example, you might repeat:

- I am kind.
- I am smart.
- I am beautiful.
- I am healthy.
- I am worthy.

Say your affirmations out loud and/or while looking in a mirror. You can also write down your affirmations or goals and post them in places where you will see them, such as on the bathroom mirror.

Mantras are statements that you repeat to yourself to achieve a sense of calm and peace. I've already shared some potential mantras in this book, including, "Think well to be well," and, "Peace begins with me." While repeating these words, it's hard to focus on any negative thoughts. Mantras make it easier to focus on the here and now, on the positive, and to live in health and wellness.

MANTRAS PRACTICE:
Nine times

- Start by finding a statement that resonates with you, such as the ones I mentioned above, or:
  - "Today is a great day."
  - "Everything is wonderful."

- Repeat your mantra nine times:
  - Three times out loud
  - Three times in a whisper
  - Three times silently in your head.

To boost the effects of your mantra, try tapping your finger to your thumb as you say each word. Some people like to use a natamala, which is sort of like a beaded necklace, although it can also be a simple string with knots. Each time you touch one of the knots, you say a word in your mantra. You become so focused touching one knot per word that it allows you to stay present. (Also, just the act of making the natamala – whether you're knotting thread or stringing beads – can be a mindful art activity, which can be done while you're in quiet thought or watching TV.)

Joe Lockett explained that he "chooses [his] thoughts, but [he] also needs to slow the process down. Once you slow life down, and it goes into slow motion, you can see what's happening, and then you can make choices."

So, by repeating mantras, we are automatically slowing ourselves down, which frees our minds to think and see more clearly. I believe that this is one of the easiest tools to learn.

JOURNALING BREAK:
Mantras

- What kind of sentences do you repeat in your head to make yourself feel better whenever you're feeling strong emotions?

- If you don't have any, think of three positive statements that you can use next time you feel this way.
- How do you think this practice will help you to calm down and feel better?

CHAKRA MEDITATION

Located along the spine, **chakras** are metaphysical energy centers that are believed to be connected to emotions, organs, health and general well-being. Although most of us cannot physically see them, we can feel their positive energy. There are seven major chakras, and each one is connected to a specific color of the rainbow, an element, a gemstone, an emotion, an organ and a belief system. Balancing the chakra centers helps us live a happy and healthy life. We can create this balance by using yoga, breath, mantras and even simple awareness. To balance the chakra energies, we focus on affirmations, positive phrases that can be written, spoken and repeated, which help us to feel better and create a positive belief system. These energy sources can calm us or recharge us.

CHAKRA MEDITATION PRACTICE:
Balancing energy by envisioning the chakras

This is one of my sister's favorite meditations. Find a comfortable sitting position and close your eyes if you feel safe in doing so. Then, visualize different-colored lights vibrating within – the colors of each chakra – and say affirmations with each one. Repeat each affirmation twice.

***

The **red chakra** is located at the base of spine. Visualize a red light where your body meets the chair or floor. The element of this chakra is earth, and it represents grounding, stability, security and safety. It is often called the root chakra.

Red chakra affirmations:
- "I am safe."
- "Mother Earth is my home. She supports me at all times, and I am never alone."

***

The **orange chakra** is located in the lower belly. Visualize orange light around your pelvic area. This chakra's element is water, and it represents creative energy and relationships.

Orange chakra affirmations:
- "I am creative. I get along well with others."
- "I create beauty in this world by sharing my talents and believing in myself, and I connect with others."

***

The **yellow chakra** is located in the solar plexus, aka the upper abdomen. Visualize bright yellow light, like the sunshine, emanating from this area. This chakra's element is fire, and it represents putting creative energy into action, strength, trusting yourself, believing in yourself and self-confidence.

Yellow chakra affirmations:

- "I am strong. I am confident."
- "I know and love who I am at every moment. This truth can never be taken from me."

***

*The **green chakra** is located at the heart center. Visualize an emerald light around your heart and chest area. The green chakra's element is air, and it represents unconditional love, self-love and forgiveness. It also represents love, health and wellness.*

Green chakra affirmations:

- "I am love. I am healthy."
- "Love is the most important aspect in my life. I give and receive love with an open heart."

***

*The **blue chakra** is located in the center of the throat. Visualize light blue light glowing in this area. The element is ether – the air above the cloud – and it represents self-expression and speaking the truth.*

Blue chakra affirmations:

- "I am truth."
- "My words are a form of energy. I speak kindly and truthfully to maintain a positive vibration."

***

*The **dark blue/indigo chakra** is located at the third eye, which is between the eyebrows. Visualize a dark blue light between your eyes. It represents the sixth sense, as well as listening, intuition and reflection.*

Dark blue chakra affirmations:
- "I am wise. I am connected."
- "There is an intelligence that exists in this world that comes from inside each of us. I listen to my inner voice to guide me."

***

*The **purple chakra** is located at the top of the head, so it is often called the crown chakra. Visualize violet light at the top of the head. Its element is space, and it represents connection to the universe, nature and spirituality – knowing we are all one.*

Purple chakra affirmations:
- "I am light. I am goodness."
- "Everything in the universe is made of light, and I am connected to everyone and everything."

***

To finish, visualize a beautiful white light surrounding you, like a protective layer. Don't forget to breathe throughout: in for four, hold for four, out for four. And be sure to sit in present gratitude, sending love and kindness to yourself and giving thanks for taking this moment.

VISUALIZATIONS

On that note, the next time you're feeling anxious or sad, or having negative thoughts, try incorporating visualizations into a meditation. **Visualizations** help you focus on the positive, cope with stress and emotions, and find your center. You can do this practice anywhere that feels comfortable to you – you can even do it while you're sitting at your desk in school.

VISUALIZATION PRACTICE:
The door

- Find a comfortable sitting position. Notice the connection of your body to the seat or floor.
- Close your eyes if you feel comfortable doing so; or, you can focus on a spot in the room that doesn't move.
- Your hands can be on your lap, palms up, or if you're at school and you prefer them on your desk, that's okay too.
- Take deep cleansing breaths. Your belly will rise on the inhale (like when you fill up a balloon with air) and relax on the exhale. This breathing provides healing oxygen and cleanses the body and mind.
- Imagine a door in front of you that leads to a state of peace, joy and safety. It can be any color, width or style that's inviting to you.
- Go to that door and open it. Walk through your door and into a place where you feel like you can breathe freely, with no weight on your shoulders – a space that feels wonderful. Maybe it is somewhere you've been on vacation, or a place in your own home. It can be indoors or outdoors, any environment that feels right

for you. For athletes, you might even try imagining being on your favorite sports field.

- Enjoy the experience by using all your senses. What do you see? What sounds can you hear? What does it smell like? Is the air moving? Is there a breeze? Are you alone, or is someone with you – a person or a pet? This is your peaceful space to create.
- Acknowledge any thoughts that enter your mind, and then release them, letting go of worries and sadness.
- Breathe in love, hold it in your heart and exhale it to share with the world. Know that everything is okay.
- Take a deep cleansing breath and remember this feeling of calmness so that you can take it with you throughout your day, feeling centered and peaceful.
- Remember: This is your safe place, somewhere that brings you a sense of peace. Anxiety and sadness do not define or control you. You are love, strength, positivity. You are worthy.
- Take another look at your surroundings, take a deep cleansing breath, and then visualize yourself standing up and walking to the door, knowing you can come back whenever you need. When you're ready, wiggle your fingers and toes, gently open your eyes and notice how you feel.

VISUALIZATION PRACTICE:
Seeing yourself on the beach
(one of my favorites)

Visualize a beautiful beach. See the blue water, the ocean waves gently touching the shore. As you breathe in, smell the ocean air as it fills up your lungs. See yourself removing your shoes, feeling the sand under your feet, wiggling your toes, feeling the sand between your toes, noticing that you're grounded on Earth. Feel the gentle breeze and the warmth of the sun on your face, the wind in your hair, the sun warming your back. Taste the salt on your tongue. Hear the waves crashing on the shore and the birds chirping as they soar above in the blue sky. If you'd like a dog with you to pet, or a horse to ride, you can visualize that, or whatever will give you comfort and bring you peace.

If thoughts enter your mind, it's okay; acknowledge and release them. Let go of all your worries and sadness. See them floating away on the wind. Breathe in love, hold it in your heart, and exhale it to share it with the world. Know that everything is okay. If you'd like, you can use a mantra, repeating words that make you feel good, such as, "Everything is great," "I am safe," "I am strong," or "Think well to be well."

VISUALIZATION PRACTICE:
Movie theater

- Start by sitting down somewhere and closing your eyes if that makes you comfortable; otherwise, stare at a spot on the floor.
- Imagine yourself in your happy place, which may be your room, a beach, the mountains, a park, a lake or anywhere that helps you feel peaceful.
- Now, picture a big movie screen in front of you. The film that's playing is filled with things that stress you

out lately, things that overwhelm you, things that make you sad or angry.

- Sit with that for a moment; notice your breath and the tension in your body. Notice how your body feels, how your heart feels, how your mind feels.
  - Is your breathing fast or slow?
  - Are your shoulders up to your ears?
  - Are your muscles tense?
- Now, clear that movie screen and watch those stressors float away and leave, just disappear, leaving behind a blank white screen. Sit with the blank screen for a minute.
- Breathe. If thoughts enter your brain, it's okay. Acknowledge and release them, without judgment, and watch as they too disappear from the screen. It's blank again.
- Notice how you're feeling. Are you experiencing less tension or breathing slower?
- Now, fill up the screen with things that make you happy – perhaps you see your family, friends, favorite sport or hobby, a pet, a song, something that makes you smile and laugh. Just as you eat nutritiously to serve your body, you are now thinking nutritiously to serve your brain.
- Now, check in again with your body.
  - Is your breathing slower?
  - Do your shoulders have less tension? Notice how your shoulders dropped away from your ears, and how your breathing feels easier, the tension gone.
  - What would happen if you deliberately put a smile on your face?
  - How does your heart feel? Your mind?

- If you can become self-aware, then you can better respond to those emotions. Breathe for a few moments and give gratitude to the screen, knowing that you can always come back to this moment if you need.
- When you're ready, take a deep breath, and if your eyes are closed, open them. Check in and notice how you feel.

If there's not a specific place that you feel comfortable visualizing, then try focusing on colors with positive affirmations.

VISUALIZATION PRACTICE:
Colors

- Go through the colors of the rainbow, beginning with red.
- Think of something that's red, then focus on it, clearing the mind in silence.
- Next, think of something associated with that color that makes you happy or brings you peace, and develop that as an associated thought. It can be a word, a picture, a sentence, a feeling.
  - For example, "I see a red flower. The color red reminds me of love. I am safe."
- Then, move onto the next color of the rainbow, in order:
  - Orange
  - Yellow
  - Green
  - Blue
  - Indigo
  - Violet.

JOURNALING BREAK:
Peace

- What is peace to you?
- What is a quiet place you like to visit?
  - Why is this a peaceful place?
  - How does it make you feel to be in this peaceful place?
  - Use the five senses to describe how the peaceful place makes you feel:
    - What can you see?
    - What can you touch?
    - What can you hear?
    - What can you smell?
    - What can you touch?

LOVING KINDNESS FOR OURSELVES AND OTHERS

The body and mind are connected, so if we can train our brains to be happier, then we can be healthier too, both individually and as a society. Dr. Dzung Vo sees the mind and the body as one thing. He says, "It's about seeing them as one whole and bringing loving awareness to our whole self, our whole being. As a pediatrician, so many of the health issues I see in teenagers have to do with stress."

So, give yourself a break. I know it's hard for us as teens, but don't judge yourself or others. Realize that while we are all different, we are also all the same. Believe in yourself – you are capable, worthy and special! **The first step in loving others is to love yourself.**

This next practice is somewhat controversial because some people think it's rooted in religion. However, I believe that mindfulness, yoga and meditation are secular and for everyone. They are about love, peace and kindness.

LOVING KINDNESS PRACTICE:
Mantras for all beings

Breathe in love and compassion on the inhale, and breathe out whatever you feel the need to release, with love and compassion, on the exhale. Then, begin to silently repeat these mantras:

- "May all beings be peaceful and live in peace."
- "May all beings be happy."
- "May all beings be healthy."
- "May all beings be safe and free from inner and outer harm."
- "May all beings be surrounded by truth, goodness, light and positivity, forever and always."
- "May all beings be filled with love and kindness."

Then, do the same thing, but change the words "all beings" to "you."

Next, think of someone with whom you feel frustration, and send these wishes to them, spreading kindness and gaining compassion in the process.

Then, repeat it again, this time thinking about someone you love deeply.

And lastly, replace the word "you" with the word "I" and grant yourself all these wishes.

Another way to give ourselves some love and kindness is to do a heartfelt practice, in which we put our hands over our hearts, offering ourselves love.

LOVING KINDNESS PRACTICE:
Heartfelt meditation

- Make sure your feet are flat on the ground, then place your hand on your chest.
- Close your eyes or look down at a point on the ground.
- Take a couple of breaths and notice how it feels to have your hand on your chest, support yourself and hold yourself in this really simple way.
- As you do this, visualize yourself giving and receiving love, giving and receiving kindness, and giving and receiving peace.
- If any thoughts arise, that's okay; notice them and let them go. Then, return to breathing in and out, and feel your hand supporting you.
- Take another deep breath into your belly, let it out, and then open your eyes gently.

YOGA AND MINDFUL MOVEMENT

Yoga can help the mind and body de-stress and focus on the present. Of course, physical health is an important component of mindfulness. Plus, when we practice mindful movement and breathing, our lymphatic system drains, and this process helps to keep us healthy. Yoga is often seen as a purely physical activity to increase flexibility and endurance, and although that is an element of the practice, it's much more than that. The true practice of yoga is bringing it off the mat and into the world. Thinking like a yogi is an integral part of living in health and happiness. It also stimulates a positive body image, generates self-confidence and increases compassion for ourselves and others.

One of the easiest ways to teach children about mindfulness is through yoga. On the mat, they can pretend to be animals, such as cows, deer, monkeys, dolphins, lions and dogs, all while making silly animal noises.

But behind all this fun, each pose has its own benefits for the body and mind. For example, dolphin pose is a great pose to strengthen the back, shoulders, arms and legs, and it also helps with balance and inner peace; calming the mind; improving coordination, focus and digestion; and relieving stress. Meanwhile, deer pose helps strengthen the spine, ribs, hips and upper legs, and it also promotes the release of negativity and focus on the positive. Downward dog pose helps energize the body and instill it with calmness, while also stretching the back, shoulders, sides and legs. As kids get older, yoga becomes a quieter and more introspective practice.

Jordan Temeres, who attended Marjory Stoneman Douglas High School, credited yoga for helping him deal with the stress and trauma of the school shooting that occurred there in February 2017. Jordan said that he's a fan of yoga, so he does a lot of it. His practice helps him by calming him and allowing him to get into the mindset of simply being comfortable.

Todd Wolfenberg says, "Yoga has an effect on the body and the mind. Yoga and meditation are about self-understanding. If you have a better understanding of yourself, then you will be a little better prepared to deal with things when they come up." That explains why yoga helped Jordan cope in the aftermath of the MSD tragedy.

MINDFUL MOVEMENT PRACTICE:
Bird-soaring breath

- Breathe in and raise your arms up to your side, then over your head.
- Exhale while floating your arms gently back down to your sides.
- Repeat.

Balance work can train the brain. We do not have to be experts at yoga to feel the benefits. A mindful movement can help us pause and be present, clearing our mind.

MINDFUL MOVEMENT PRACTICE:
Building on a simple stretch

One simple movement to try is raising your arms above your head with your palms touching, taking a deep breath in and stretching to the right side.

From there, release a breath, return to center and do the same thing on the left side. The stretch feels good for the body, and the mind benefits too.

If you would like to add something to this movement, then bend your knee and lift your leg, placing your foot on the inner thigh of the standing leg.

Now, you can visualize being a tree with your branches blowing in the wind. Keep your eyes on something in front of you that's not moving – that will help you balance.

Remember to breathe, and whatever you do on one side, you must then do on the other side as well. So, if you balance on your left foot, be sure to do the same on your right foot. Try flowing through this pose and see if you notice a difference in how you feel.

> **"If every child in the world is taught meditation, we would eliminate violence within one generation."**
> **– The Dalai Lama**

MEDITATION

The Dalai Lama said, "If every child in the world is taught meditation, we would eliminate violence within one generation."[33] We need to be teaching meditation to help the next generation cope better.

Meditation means being in quiet thought and stillness, allowing the active thinking mind to settle inward, and thus experiencing a calm, peaceful level of awareness. Meditation increases attention and lowers anxiety and depression. Bob Roth says, "Meditation, for me, in those choppy waves, drops an anchor. It's like I've got some inner stability. I'm not overreacting, I'm not a victim. I'm stronger than that. I handle that. It keeps me calm inside and wakes up my brain so I can focus better. Meditation is a natural antidote that makes you feel happier inside."

Madison McEvoy, another student from MSD in Parkland, agrees. She meditates a lot because "meditation helps clear the mind instead of focusing on everything going on in the world, which would drive you crazy."

I can relate to that. If I let my mind go all over the place, I would probably be upset, anxious, angry or sad more often.

Holding on to feelings like that can lead us to lash out at our parents or get into arguments with friends that make us feel awful afterward. If we are taught mindfulness or meditation, these tools become automatic responses to daily stress, and we will grow up to be less depressed and anxious; instead, we will be happier, more content, peace-loving adults.

Learning mindfulness is a little harder once you become a teenager, but only because your coping mechanisms and how you deal with stress and make choices have become habitual by then.

But you can form new healthier habits by practicing meditation. Todd Wolfenberg explains that "meditation trains [your] mind, helps you become better at observing what's going on, and allows thinking and feeling without having to react all the time." There is freedom in learning how to take a step back. It gives you choice.

I attended a workshop with Jon Kabat-Zinn, widely known as the Father of Mindfulness. When he was talking about the benefits of meditation, he said something that made me pause: "Some people say they fall asleep when they meditate. I like to say I fall awake. We have a liberative choice."[34] My interpretation of what he said is this: If you take the time to clear your mind, then you're able to reel yourself in, gain clarity and realize what truly matters in life. Once you achieve that, you can live in gratitude and wellness, have more patience with yourself and others, and know how you want to contribute to the world. Your problems may not seem insurmountable any longer, and you may attain some semblance of inner peace, understanding and recognition that it was right there in front of you, for you to grab, the entire time. Want to feel all of the above? A body scan is a good place to start.

MEDITATION PRACTICE:
Body scan

- Sit comfortably with your hands on your lap and your feet grounded on the floor, if you are in a chair.
- Check in with yourself: How does your body feel? Do you feel relaxed? How does your mind feel? How are you feeling overall today? What's on your mind? Notice any urges to move or shift. Notice any area of tension.
- Continue to breathe in and out mindfully, with your eyes closed if that's comfortable for you; otherwise, focus on a place on the floor. As you inhale, remember that mindful breathing strengthens the diaphragm and provides oxygen to all of your organs.
- Bring your attention down to the toes of your right foot. Notice the top of your right foot, the bottom, the heel. Move your attention up to your ankle, lower leg and calf muscle. Then, draw your focus up to your knee, thigh, hamstring and quadricep muscles. Hold your entire right foot and leg in your awareness. Notice the support it provides.
- As you move up to your right hip, move across to your left hip, and then bring your attention down to the tips of your toes on your left foot, and do the same thing on the left side.
- Check in with yourself and see how you're doing now, if there are any feelings that are present.
- Breathe into any areas where you find discomfort and gently, slowly release that breath.
- When thoughts come, remember that it's natural to have thoughts. Acknowledge them, release them without judgment and come back to the present.

- Move your attention up to your stomach, keeping your hand there so you can feel the belly rising on the in-breath and gently falling on the out-breath. Your lungs and ribs also expand and contract as you breathe. Notice how your breath grounds you to the present moment, free from the past or future, allowing you to be here, now.
- As you move up your chest, bring awareness to your heart. Tune into its beating, notice the support it provides and send gratitude for that support. Do the same for your lungs before you move up to your collarbone, then to the right side of your right shoulder, bringing your attention down to the tips of your fingers on your right hand.
- Move up to your wrist and forearm, your elbow, biceps and triceps. Bring your awareness to your entire right hand and arm.
- As you reach your shoulder, bring your attention across your collarbone to the left side of your shoulder and left arm, doing the same thing on the left side.
- Now, notice both hands and arms, and breathe into any areas of discomfort. Notice what you feel and what's present there.
- As you move up to your shoulders, bring your attention down to the lower back, the bottom of your spine, all the way up the top of your back, your neck and then to your cervical spine. Breathe into your back, sending breath to any area of discomfort. Notice the support your back provides, sending gratitude for that support.
- Bring your attention to your shoulders. Release any tension, bringing your shoulders away from your ears.

- Notice your neck and the back of your head, moving to your forehead and the front of your face. Let go of any facial expression you might be holding. Notice your forehead and temples, as well as your eyes, cheeks and nose.
- Notice your jaw, and if it's clenched, release it. Notice your ears and mouth, dropping your tongue if it's on the roof of your mouth.
- Bring awareness to your breath. Let it be your anchor. Notice your chin and throat, and the movement of breath in your lungs and stomach. Holding your entire body in awareness, breathe beautiful light and oxygen into any areas you wish. Let go of anything that doesn't serve you.
- Remember to breathe in love and goodness on the inhale, and release negativity on the exhale. Or, if you feel comfortable, breathe in love for your family, yourself and the world, and then breathe out love for your family, yourself and the world.
- Know that you can take a piece of how you feel to the rest of your day if you choose. When you're ready to gently let awareness of your surroundings come back, you can send a note of gratitude to the universe.
- Slowly wiggle your fingers and toes, roll your neck to one side and then the other. Then, take a deep cleansing breath, release it and open your eyes, coming back to the room, noticing how you feel.

When I do this practice, I like to imagine healing, protective white light surrounding and filling up my body as I perform the scan.

SELF-REFLECTION

You've already seen many self-reflection prompts throughout this book. You can always take a few quiet moments to check in with yourself, breathe and see how you're feeling. If you've already tried answering some of these prompts, then you know how good it feels to sit in a peaceful environment or quiet the mind with journaling. After Grandpa died, my mom dealt with her grief by writing to him in a journal, which helped her a lot because it made her feel like she was still able to tell him things. Once again, the goal here is not to stop the mind from wandering, but to acknowledge, release without judgment and consider each moment as a new opportunity.

> **"Let it go. No amount of worrying about it is going to change things."**
>
> **– Jennifer Miller**

Jennifer Miller says that "it's hard to get off the hamster wheel, but it goes nowhere. Those negative thoughts aren't constructive. Recognize that you're stewing on something negative, and either talk to a friend about it or write it in a journal and get it out. Ask, 'How can I see this in another way, and how can I set a positive goal?' And then let it go. No amount of worrying about it is going to change things."

JOURNALING

On that note, journaling helps you figure things out and let them go. You can write about what stresses you out, what makes you flip out, how you handle your fight/flight/freeze instincts, and whether you can choose a more mindful solution to your problems. If you can name your feelings, you can breathe through them and take full responsibility for yourself and your actions. You can make better choices if you understand what drives you.

Have you ever thought or said something you've later come to regret? I think we all have. Journaling about your feelings can offer you some perspective, understanding, acceptance and self-compassion. You can journal about how your day went or a specific event that occurred, processing your emotions in a healthy way.

If sitting down with a pen and paper isn't for you, then you can always take notes on your phone about what you're feeling and why. There are also lots of books with specific prompts for journaling to help you get started. Identifying your feelings is a really big deal because it's a path to healing, in that you're giving yourself permission to be human, acknowledging your emotions and missteps, and coming up with ways to handle them better, whether that's now or in the future.

JOURNALING BREAK:
The story of you

Write a chapter in the story of you: a time that stressed you out, and how you coped with the stress. In hindsight, how could you have dealt with the emotion in a positive way?

REFLECTION

If you don't have a journal handy, you can also reflect on things in the moment before speaking. Wuf Shanti teaches the **THINK** acronym:

- Is it True?
- Is it Helpful?
- Is it Inspiring?
- Is it Necessary?
- Is it Kind?

Dr. Dzung Vo likes the **STOP** method:

- Stop what you're doing or what you were about to do.
- Take three mindful breaths.
- Observe what's happening in the present moment, and then
- Proceed with awareness and kindness, choosing what you want to do based on what's going to be the most helpful for yourself and others.

JOURNALING BREAK:
Pause

- Consider a time when someone said something that hurt your feelings.
  - Do you think the person who said it used the THINK technique first?
  - How could that person have spoken differently if they thought before they spoke?
  - If they had used the THINK technique, how would that have made you feel?
- What are your personal pausing techniques?
- Do you believe that practicing a behavior can change the brain, and positive actions can become habitual? Why or why not?
- Write about a time that you reacted without pausing and how the outcome could have been different if you used the STOP technique.

"Ask yourself this question: Is this useful? It can help you draw the line between useless rumination and constructive anguish."

– Dan Harris

When it comes to in-the-moment reflecting, Dan Harris simply likes to ask if things are useful. He says, "When you notice that you're in a loop of negative thinking on something, like a test score, fight with a friend, some new rule your parents introduced around the house that you don't like, maybe ask yourself this question: Is this useful? It can help you draw the line between useless rumination and constructive anguish. That's a huge deal... There's a way through, developing self-awareness and mindfulness to notice when you've worried yourself silly, it's no longer useful and maybe it's time to do something else." I like this form of self-reflection because it helps me put things into perspective. If it's not going to be important in a few weeks, then maybe I can let it go.

GETTING OUTSIDE

This may not seem like a traditional mindfulness practice, but it's vital – so many of us who were stuck indoors due to Covid can attest to that. Try going outside and breathing some fresh air, even if it's just for a minute. Or, you can spend more time outside and take a walk around the block, ride a bike, play an individual sport. I like to play golf or shoot hoops. My sister likes to swim. Just as with the long list of mindful practices, find the one that works for you.

MOVEMENT PRACTICE:
Walking to feel good

Walking around silently lets us focus on things we don't usually see or hear. Try it:
- Quietly and calmly walk in silence, breathing the air, noticing what you see and observe while on the walk.

- Remember to breathe as you are looking around and appreciating your surroundings.
- You can make your walk even more mindful by choosing a color or shape to look for, then counting in your head the number of times that you see it.

"There are so many tools to put in your toolbox, and you have to find which works for you."

– Ross Robinson

MINDFUL WRAP-UP

As Ross Robinson of the Holistic Life Foundation notes, "There are so many tools to put in your toolbox, and you have to find which works for you." For example, Ross likes to practice positive thinking because then positivity gravitates back toward him. But, as he says, you need to figure out which practices you enjoy – and make you more mindful in the process. Meditation can help you stay calm and focused. Even spending time with animals might be a source of calm for you. Talking to someone you trust is super healthy too. Remember: Self-regulation and stress reduction can both be learned.

Best of all, we can get a handle on our emotions and practice responding instead of reacting. We can reply with love.

JOURNALING BREAK:
Self-reflection

Pick two of the following to write about in your journal today:
- What gets you into a bad mood, and what can get you out of it?

- When you want to talk to your best friend, what is your favorite method of communication? Why?
- What are your biggest day-to-day worries and stressors?
- How do you usually deal with these stressors or solve problems?
- How do you usually calm yourself down when you are upset?

Who's your favorite celebrity? Chances are, they have adopted a mindful practice – and they have made a point to share it, too.

There are so many celebrities who are starting to talk about their mental health and/or the mindful practices that help them de-stress, which is also great for teens to hear because they pay attention to people they look up to and admire. For example, according to Adam Levine of Maroon 5, "Yoga welcomes everyone… it has given me the ability to be more focused and make better decisions… and teaches us to be still and calm under challenging circumstances."[35] Other well-known people who practice some form of yoga, meditation or mindfulness include Lady Gaga, Ahmir "Questlove" Thompson, Justin Timberlake, Oprah Winfrey and Gwyneth Paltrow. Take a cue from your role models who are practicing mindfulness daily.

Mindfulness matters. And training your mind needs to be learned, just like math and science. You don't automatically know how to communicate with others, handle stress or emotions, live a healthy lifestyle or show kindness. We need to feel our emotions, but we also need to learn how to process them in a healthy way. It's about recognizing those emotions, accepting and regulating them, and releasing them. This journey, if you decide to take it, will require compassion and empathy for yourself and others.

11

AUTHENTIC CONNECTION

From Communication to Inclusion to Empathy

I have long believed that we need to teach kids and teens about diversity and inclusion – that's why the first Wuf Shanti song I ever wrote with my dad was called "Let's Dance Together." Learning these things is a direct path to compassion and empathy.

Teens have an internal battle with self-esteem and self-confidence, made worse by social media. Instead of thinking, "I'm not good enough," and comparing yourself to others, you can develop a greater sense of self-worth, appreciate others' differences and also welcome the similarities of a common humanity. If you want to face these challenges, authenticity is key; learning emotional intelligence, purpose and self-love are integral to finding yourself – and being confident in who you are.

> **"We get in trouble when we hold things in. When we communicate, we are healthier."**
>
> **– Dan Devone**

COMMUNICATION

Mindfulness can help us learn how to communicate and resolve conflicts, love others and likewise love ourselves in the process. Dan Devone told me, "We get in trouble when we hold things in.

When we communicate, we are healthier. If you're constantly talking about how you feel or what's going on in your life, that's the healthiest person in the room. Those are the people that are going to be well adjusted. All of us need an opportunity just to talk to somebody. The ability to talk to other people and flush things out of your head – it's healthy for all of us, so keep the lines of communication open and talk, talk, talk!"

One technique we use with preteens is the talking stick, or peace wand. Whoever is holding it has the right to speak while everyone else listens. They can also make the talking sticks themselves. It is a mindful art activity, which can then be used for making introductions, having quiet time, sharing exciting news or talking about what is making them happy or sad. Most importantly, anyone with the talking stick learns the three keys to effective communication:

- Speaking from the heart
- Speaking respectfully and with kindness
- Active listening.

Teens don't really have an equivalent to a talking stick, but we can still learn to communicate well. All we need is a shift in perspective, which we can gain if we set our intention to listen to each other mindfully.

According to Dr. Amy Saltzman, "We can stop and breathe and choose to really hear our own truths, and then hear the other person's truths. Usually, when your parents are on you about something, at the bottom is fear. They are worried about you because they love you. They are scared. Say, 'Dad/Mom, I understand you love me, and I understand you're worried, and it's all going to be fine,' and that will change the conversation." Imagine if we tried that instead of immediately playing defense – it would help us all to have less contentious relationships with our parents.

> **"If people really stopped and paused and asked what the other person is feeling, it would open the door to understanding another person better."**
> **– Dave Trachtenberg**

ASKING QUESTIONS

On that note, to better understand where someone is coming from – and to better understand ourselves – asking questions can be even more helpful than pausing or breathing.

Supna Shah says that most people, including teens, "are usually already preparing our answer before we've even heard what the person has said. The best tool for nurturing self-awareness is asking questions. Anxiety and depression are a pattern of choice in behavior that we can change, so when we start to feel this stress, it's our responsibility to ourselves to ask what's causing it, and what we are going to consciously decide to do about it."

JOURNALING BREAK:
Listening and asking questions

- Why do you think we should ask each other questions about ourselves?
- What does empathy mean to you? What does diversity and inclusion mean to you?
- Is it important to be able to recognize the perspective of others? Why or why not?
- Think of a difficult situation you're in or that you've gone through recently. Put yourself in the shoes of someone you admire and ask yourself how they would deal with it.

- Consider the last argument you had with someone, and then switch sides. Write about it from the other person's perspective. Has this changed your point of view?

Learning to ask questions with curiosity – whether we're speaking to ourselves or others – is a technique that can generate kindness and compassion, which are strengths that empower us to face and overcome challenges to change our lives in a positive way. Walk the Middle Way's Dave Trachtenberg encourages teens to "ask ourselves questions like, 'How am I feeling now?' 'What would I like to be feeling now if I'm stressed?' 'Where is peace for me right now?' Questions lead to greater awareness. Then, we should ask others these questions, too. If people really stopped and paused and asked what the other person is feeling, it would open the door to understanding another person better, and that's the first step."

ACTIVE LISTENING PRACTICE:
Look within

For ten minutes, set aside time to listen to yourself.
- Notice what you see, hear and feel as you simply sit or walk in silence without being connected to any technology.
- Notice any random thoughts that come into your head.
- Afterward, sort the thoughts into categories of things that are facts/known, and things that are opinions or possibilities.
- Ask yourself a different question each day and sit in honesty with the answer.

CREATING AN OPEN DIALOGUE

Listening is just part of the puzzle. We can't reach internal peace nor world peace if we don't have an open dialogue with each other, either. As teen Madison McEvoy told me, "I think as long as we all work together and communicate nicely and figure out how we can work on things together, then the world will be a better place. We don't have to agree on everything – we can agree to disagree and still work on things."

The first thing we need to do, though, is put the phones down and talk to each other for real. We think we are more connected than ever, but really, we are more disconnected than ever. Dan Devone said during our interview that he's "not telling teens to throw their phones in the ocean. I'm attached to my phone like everyone else, but what I encourage is a sense of balance. If your desk is two feet to the right of mine, how about turning in your chair and speaking with me face to face, instead of texting me? There used to be a time that people walked down the street and said hello to each other, and now, I'd settle for a head nod if people could just look up from their phones. It's important for us to have a balance and connect with other people in the world so that we can be healthier." That's a really good point about texting. How many times have you been at the same table or in the same room as someone and texted them instead of talking face to face?

Dr. Chris Willard agrees. He said, "When one person pulls out their phone, everyone else does it. It's contagious, like yawning. It's not easy for anyone, even adults. If you're out to dinner, and even one person has their phone out on the table, it reduces conversation by 30 percent. Keep it in your bag or a drawer so it doesn't tempt you. That can help with the addictive nature."

"Look up – life is happening."

– Cory Alexander

I know it annoys my parents when I'm looking at my phone while having a conversation with them. I used to justify it by saying that I was capable of doing two things at once. But actually, that's not really the point. As Cory Alexander puts it, "Where you are, let your whole self be there and engage. Look up – life is happening. If you're out with friends, and everyone is on their phones, they aren't appreciating the fellowship. If you can't see someone is upset, then you can't say to yourself, 'Maybe I should be more compassionate.'" Human connection and interaction are keys to our well-being.

Consider this:

The next time someone texts you, call them. Better yet, FaceTime them.

My Grandpa Alan used to tell me to take some time at the end of every day and call someone who I hadn't spoken to in a while, just to say hi and check in, to let them know that I was thinking of them. I never really understood how that was different from texting until the Covid-19 pandemic kept us all apart. Consider how you'd feel if someone made an effort to call you just to ask how you are. Wouldn't you feel appreciated? Like you're not taken for granted? Like someone out there actually cares about you? Now, extend that to others. As teen Elayna Hasty said, "Love yourself, but also love those around you. Be good to yourself and be good to others. You never know what they're going through unless you're in their shoes." What if they are having an exceptionally rough time, and hearing your voice and seeing your face actually lets them know that they can talk to you? I know that we are all super busy with school and life, but what's a few minutes to let someone know you're there for them?

I now always try to make time to speak to people. And if they call me, and for some reason I can't get to the phone, I always make it a point to return the call the same day. Here's another tip from Grandpa Alan, and this one can help you one day in your career, too: Clients will appreciate that you are accessible, that you care enough about them to take time out of your day to return the call and give them your undivided attention. Replace the word "clients" with "friends," and the advice still stands!

COMMUNICATING WITH YOURSELF

Matt Dewar said, "When do you feel and do your best? For most people, it's when we are consciously connected. Mindfulness is remembering to come back to what's most important, which is the life that's right at our fingertips."

To that end, the way we communicate with ourselves and with others is essential, too. Matt suggests that teens "take a week, get a notepad, carry it around and write down your thoughts throughout the day. You will distill all your thoughts down to a few that dictate the inner workings of your mind. Often, with many people, a lack of self-worth is a really common driving thought. All of your thoughts will come from that core belief lens, and your actions will come from that. If you can start to identify and record your patterns of thinking, core thoughts and core beliefs, you can start to question them and work with them."

Therefore, the manner in which we talk to ourselves can have an impact on our self-confidence and self-esteem, and vice versa, our self-esteem and self-confidence can have an impact on how we communicate with ourselves and others, leading either to conflict or healthy relationships.

As Amy Eva of the Greater Good Science Center told me, "It's really important to think about how your thoughts and feelings affect your behavior. Eighty percent of us treat others better than we treat ourselves. It's really important to have skills that will help you to be kinder to yourself. One easy thing we can do to boost our self-esteem and self-confidence is to repeat affirmations." I wrote about affirmations earlier, but let's try a practice now because affirmations help us reduce our anxiety, cope with emotions, and perceive and treat ourselves and others with more kindness.

COMMUNICATING WITH YOURSELF:
Self-esteem

- Consider your limiting self-beliefs. For example:
  - "I am not good enough."
  - "I am not lovable."
- Ask where that limiting self-belief lives in the body (stomach, chest, throat). Does it have a shape, a color, an image?
- Reverse the belief verbally:
  - "I AM good enough."
  - "I AM lovable."
- Where does the positive belief reside? What's its color, shape, image, place in the body?
- Visualize living the positive belief, and how your life, home, school and friendships would be if you did.
- Say your positive affirmations out loud, and then have a trusted friend repeat them back to you: "You are good enough."

JOURNALING BREAK:
Positivity

- Write down ten positive things about yourself that start with "I AM."

One of my friends, Clair, has panic attacks, almost to the point of making her agoraphobic (and they started before Covid made us wary of crowds.) Affirmations are what gets her through them. I rely on affirmations too. I like to say something positive in the mornings to start the day off right, like "Today is a good day," or when things are going rough at any point during the day, I say something like "Everything is okay."

As I previously mentioned, affirmations can be said silently to yourself, or you can stick post-it notes up around the house or on the bathroom mirror so that these statements are the first thing you see as you get ready in the morning – and the last thing you see as you get ready for bed. And even better, you'll see yourself in the mirror at the same time that you see and say these positive statements, thereby associating them with yourself in your mind. If you see and say them often enough, they will eventually become part of who you are, and you will believe them. This can make a huge change for teens because some of us are really hard on ourselves, and it's good to know that we're all deserving of love.

COMMUNICATING WITH YOURSELF:
Affirmations

Here are some examples of affirmations for you to try out:
- "I am safe."
- "I am healthy."
- "I am grateful."
- "I am smart."
- "I am kind."
- "I am special."
- "I am worthy."

Learning to speak to yourself with kindness not only generates self-confidence, but also allows you to accept yourself, believe in yourself, have self-compassion and live authentically. In fact, J.G. Larochette believes authenticity is key. "There has to be a real connection with the self, self-love and self-compassion. We aren't our emotions and negative thoughts. Often, we attach to our thoughts and emotions, and we get stuck in a cycle of self-criticism and beating ourselves up. We need to give ourselves permission to BE, without judgment. We need to rewire ourselves to accept that we are each special, our uniqueness is what we need to show, and we only need to fit into our own well-being. We need to not believe these messages that society is sending us and stay true to who we are."

Think about it like this: If someone has a negative self-image or a lack of self-esteem, then they may be more likely to struggle with life's ups and downs, buckle under stress or live a life of addiction, and they may not develop loving relationships or allow themselves to become their true selves.

One of my friends, Kelly, believed what some of the girls in class were saying about her and became especially hard on herself – so hard on herself that she developed an eating disorder. Affirmations would not have solved all her problems, but maybe if she had learned some mindful techniques (like affirmations) to help boost her self-esteem and realize that she is a great human being, she would have had a better time dealing with the situation.

"You can't go anywhere else in the world and find another you. You have to stop and understand how truly special and unique you are."
– Sadiqa Glusman

Ross Robinson had a really good point about this. He said, "Self-love is so empowering. No one else controls it. It's a gift that you and only you can control. The world is going to be crazy, so anchor yourself down. *Life is the waves. Your breath can be your anchor.*" And as Sadiqa Glusman said, "You can't go anywhere else in the world and find another you. You have to stop and understand how truly special and unique you are. When you start to see yourself as special and unique, you'll stop doing destructive things. Find your worth and shine."

YOUR TRUE SELF

Once you learn that you are special, accept yourself the way you are and start to be true to yourself, then you can then help others. All of this – self-esteem, self-confidence, self-compassion, authenticity and communication – brings you closer to others and gives you a greater understanding, compassion and empathy for what others are going through. Whitney Stewart says, "If we believe we are okay – and even wonderful – just the way we are, show ourselves deep compassion, and then share that compassion and respect for others who are probably going through similar situations, we can find our inner strength, develop a better relationship with ourselves and a better relationship with others."

MINDFUL ART PRACTICE:
Mindful Me Tree

Sadiqa Glusman first introduced me to the Mindful Me Tree, also called a self-awareness tree, and it's a super simple and eye-opening mindful art activity.

- Draw a big tree, from the roots to the trunks to the branches.

- On the roots, write what you're good at that no one can take away from you (e.g., "I am good at writing," "I am good at caring," "I am good at baking," etc.).
- In the middle of the tree – its trunk – put your strengths that help you get out of a black hole when you make a conscious decision to do so (e.g., "I am a good friend," "I am a hard worker," "I am kind," "I am helpful," etc.).
- At the top of the tree – along the branches and within the leaves – are your goals and what you want to accomplish (e.g., "I want to be a good person who makes a difference in the world," "I want to be a veterinarian that helps heal animals," etc.).

The students really appreciate this activity because it helps them "see" their true selves – and I bet you'll feel the same if you try it.

J.G. Larochette believes, "Our authentic, true self is what we need to shine a light on. There's never been another you in the world, and that's all we need. Don't feel like you have to be any different, other than what you are really about. Really align the mind, body and spirit as much as possible, and do what nourishes those three. Let go of stereotypes or conditioning and be you. Let your heart open instead of hardening. Practice as much as possible gratitude, mindfulness and self-compassion, which are the three ingredients to really being healthy in mind, body and heart." Once you accept your true self, begin to live authentically and treat yourself with kindness, then you can begin to understand, interact with and appreciate others on a higher level.

JOURNALING BREAK:
Staying true to you

- Write about a time that you felt like your true self, and how that made you feel. How do you think you could allow yourself to be your true self more often?
- Why should you be authentic?
- What happens to you when you feel uncomfortable? For example, do you giggle?
  - Why do you think you have the reaction that you have?
- Why should you be kind to yourself and others?

DIVERSITY AND INCLUSION

But to get to compassion and empathy, we must first understand diversity and inclusion. Have you ever noticed that kids don't see differences much and simply love each other? They just want to be friends and have fun together. What happens when we grow up? Why do we start judging, isolating and criticizing? And how can we get back to basics?

The best way to do that is to learn mindful communication skills, such as asking questions, and mindful observation skills, and have those as our foundation. As Dave Smith told us in Chapter 1, it's like playing basketball – we have to learn to dribble the ball first before we can make a layup.

Maureik Robison thinks we can start by mindfully listening. He once told me, "There are lots of people not listening to understand, and instead they're waiting to speak. So, they're not in the moment. When communicating between two people, it is really important to actively listen." Sadiqa Glusman agreed when I asked her about diversity and inclusion, and how to reach a place of empathy: "I'm big about asking questions and talking about the elephant in the room. After you talk about it, you feel better. I'm okay with feeling uncomfortable. It helps us be mindful."

DIVERSITY AND INCLUSION PRACTICE:
Common humanity

- Pair up with a friend and spend the next minute looking at each other in silence.
- Notice if you have different skin colors, as well as the shapes of your eyes, the textures of your hair, your noses, mouths, if you are each tall or short, etc.
- Now, think about what you have in common, things are similar about you both.
  ○ We've all felt happiness; we've all felt sadness; we've all had accomplishments; we've all experienced pain; we've all experienced fear; we all have a heart, etc.
- Now, close your eyes and picture the other person, wishing them health, strength, joy, peace, etc.
- When you open your eyes, give gratitude to the other person for sharing this experience with you.

We teach this common humanity practice often through Wuf Shanti, and sometimes it makes the students uncomfortable; however, hands down, every single person who has done it has appreciated it and the lessons they learned.

I remember doing this practice at a high school once, and there were two girls in the front row who started crying. When I asked why, they explained that by looking into each other's eyes, they actually *saw* each other and understood what the other person had gone through. They didn't know any of the details or specifics, but they knew they both had experienced great joy and great pain in their lives, a shared humanity. This five-minute practice changed their perceptions of each other and, I'd venture to say, their outlooks on life. A humanity practice is a good teaching tool to start on the road to acceptance and empathy.

Common humanity practices like these not only teach the participants to accept without judgment and to recognize a common humanity, which leads to an understanding of diversity, inclusion, compassion and empathy; but it also teaches the students about themselves. Dr. Regina Washington, formerly of CenterLink: The Community of LGBT Centers, says, "Diversity starts with the self. You, as a person, have different experiences, likes, dislikes. Appreciate what you bring to the table and appreciate others around you. Take a moment to learn about yourself and others."

At the end of the common humanity practice, we often ask the teens to raise a hand if they felt uncomfortable looking into each other's eyes in silence. A majority of students inevitably raise their hands. We ask them to look within and ask themselves why – what thoughts were going through their heads? Were they judging, comparing or being self-critical, or were they thinking about the party they want to go to on the weekend or the argument they had with someone earlier that day? We also ask them to acknowledge how the feeling of being uncomfortable manifested itself physically. This allows them to understand how they react to different situations. The majority of students will say they started laughing, which tells them that when they feel nervous, they tend to laugh, and that's a good thing to know about oneself.

JOURNALING BREAK:
We are all one

- What preconceived opinions do you have about other people?
- Where do you think bias comes from? Are you capable of seeing beyond the cover, accepting in a nonjudgmental way?
- Have you ever found a connection with someone who looked or sounded different from you? Write about that experience.
- What are your thoughts and feelings about helping others? How about asking for help when you need it?
- Should you help a new student? How would you feel if you were new? How could you help a new student? What would you want people to do for you?

Because I think this is such a vital topic, I want to share a few more enlightening practices from Helen Maffini of Mind-Be Education.

DIVERSITY AND INCLUSION PRACTICE:
In their shoes

In this exercise, students imagine what it is like to be the character in a book, such as Scout in *To Kill a Mockingbird*, and they "explore how that character might feel, see and do things, and the reasons why they made the choices they made, and if the students would have felt the same way or handled the situation the same way."

DIVERSITY AND INCLUSION PRACTICE:
Perspective cards

With "perspective" situation cards, students explore how the same situation might be viewed in different ways by different people.

According to Helen, these practices "help everyone to realize that sometimes, no one is wrong; it is just how they witnessed certain things. We work from there to discuss and see how we can be empathetic to others." These practices can be done on your own, observing, asking questions, looking at things from different perspectives. The next time you read a book or disagree with something that someone says, think about this idea and give it a try – put yourself in their shoes and see if it offers you a better understanding.

> **"Communication is a good springboard for diversity and inclusion."**
> **– Dr. Regina Washington**

Dr. Regina Washington also believes that mindful communication practices lead to improvements in inclusiveness. She says, "Once you teach people how to ask questions [...], how to communicate with people who are different than they are and how to listen, that can be transformed into application. Communication is a good springboard for diversity and inclusion." This is why Wuf

Shanti will often do a mindful communication with teens. We have them practice asking each other questions about their backgrounds, cultures, nationalities, customs and more. Then, the next day, we provide hypotheticals, and they role-play various scenarios, like how to discuss difficult topics and handle conflict in a peaceful manner.

THE POSSE FOUNDATION

Leading up to college, I was accepted as a Posse Scholar in the Posse Foundation. Posse is an organization that focuses on leadership, diversity and inclusion, and selects ten kids who have made an impact on the world to attend college together. It's a built-in support system at college, and for me, that's the best part. When I met my Posse, we instantly connected and became really good friends. I think the reason we got along so well was because, even though we come from different cultures and places, we had a common goal to make the world better.

Every week, our group meets for a workshop to discuss a different topic, such as culture, politics, religion, gender/sexuality, communication skills and more. A big part of each discussion is going around the room and asking difficult questions and listening to the answers in a respectful manner. Through this process, I've learned different viewpoints and ideas that I might not have considered without being exposed to this group.

Before these discussions, I may not have taken the time to ask questions if dealing with someone who had a different philosophy. I may have inadvertently made a mistake in something I said. Now, I know to ask questions because even if I disagree with someone's viewpoint, I can have a better understanding of where they are coming from. Only with active listening and authentic communication can we bridge the divide that is happening in our country – and divides happening across the world.

I'm sure there will be times that I say or do something that, upon reflection, I won't be proud of, but I'm going to try to give myself a break because hindsight is 20/20. I will try to learn from the experience and not make the same mistake again. My hope is to always try to build bridges, to get people with different perspectives and beliefs to be kind to each other and work together for the common good. Maybe this is something that comes with life experiences.

JOURNALING BREAK:
Learning lessons

Write about a time that you did something with good intentions but came to realize that you may have unintentionally hurt people.
- What lesson did you learn?
- How will you handle the situation differently next time?
- Can you offer yourself some forgiveness and compassion? How?

As I've said so many times before, learning perspective, acceptance, empathy and how to love ourselves and others are keys to mindfulness.

Volunteering is another way for teens to learn all of these things by getting to know those who live differently than they do. Helen Maffini says we should "encourage students to volunteer and, if possible, for classes to do so together. Working in a food kitchen or handing out packages to homeless individuals can help us develop empathy and understanding." In my school, we have a Best Buddy program that teaches acceptance and empathy because it shares with teens how to be inclusive of those with intellectual and developmental disabilities and treat them with kindness and respect, as they would want to be treated. Any form of volunteering you want to take on will do. That's because, as Dr. Sam Himmelstein shared with me, "It's not really the technique – it's the humanity between us and the authenticity in the relationship. It's amazing what people will do if you [...] build a real relationship with them. It's the core element of the work."

12

IMPROVING OUR RELATIONSHIPS

Compassion, Connection and Collaboration

Argos Gonzalez of Little Flower Yoga believes that when "we take three breaths, we're showing ourselves lots of compassion and taking care of ourselves, and we all need that. The more we take care of ourselves, being compassionate toward ourselves, the easier it is to be compassionate with others." He sees a link "between taking those three breaths and making the world a better place. It's not going solve all your problems but it will help you deal with whatever arises a little bit more skillfully."

Mindfulness-based social-emotional learning (MBSEL) skills are not only about regulating and healing yourself, but also about how to best interact with others. By learning these techniques, you can better connect with others, not only to be able to collaborate, but also to experience empathy.

EMPATHY

Supna Shah defines empathy as "putting yourself in someone else's shoes. It's so important and can change the world because when we connect on a human level – person to person, in person – it's a whole different level of connection and understanding of someone else's life experiences, and it puts both of our lives in perspective. It reminds us that we're all connected and 99 percent the same." This is the path to a more peaceful world. Can you imagine if our ancestors had learned this way back when? Maybe there wouldn't have been wars, famine, bullying or isolation. And maybe we wouldn't have such high levels of illness, self-harm or harm to others. Thinking positively is important, for sure, but to me, empathy is one of the biggest secrets to living mindfully.

As Dave Trachtenberg stated, "Empathy affects everything else like mindfulness and diversity and inclusion. We need to ask ourselves what it's like to walk in the shoes of other people and see from their perspective what their experience is and what they're going through." One meme I saw showed humans on the top saying that 2020 was the worst year of their lives, and then it showed dogs on the bottom saying that 2020 was the best year of their lives because their humans spent every minute with them. Perspective.

In school, I read the book *Black Like Me* by John Howard Griffin, which was published in 1961. The book tells the story of how the white author decided to walk in the shoes of a Black man in the Deep South in the 1960s. In the book, Mr. Griffin takes pills to turn his skin darker, and then goes out into the world to see how people treat him.[36] While I do not think we should need to change our appearance to learn empathy, it was an interesting lesson in how we see each other, treat each other and connect with each other.

Of course, reading is not the only way to gain an understanding of what someone has been through. In fact, to gain a better understanding of others, I propose we start here:

WE CAN TALK TO EACH OTHER

Once again, communication is key. Supna Shah urges us to "have the uncomfortable conversations. Talk about our emotions and feelings. Ask questions and actively listen." And teen Sophie Riegel shares that "to help a loved one dealing with a mental health condition, ask them what you can do for them at the moment because it's not about you, it's about them. Don't try to make someone dealing with anxiety or depression feel something other than what they're feeling. Just be there with them in the moment. Say something like, 'This must be really hard for you. Tell me more about that.'" I've learned not to tell anyone to "stop feeling" what they are feeling or to "calm down" or that they "are okay." Instead, I tell them it's okay to feel what they are feeling, and I ask questions like, "How can I help you?"

COMMUNICATION PRACTICE:
Paraphrasing

- Put down your phone for a bit and have an actual conversation with your parents or a friend.
- Ask how they are, listen to the answer and then paraphrase it back to them.
- Allow them to ask you questions, too, and look them in the eyes while you answer.
- Notice how you feel, and if you feel heard.

WE CAN MEET IN THE MIDDLE

Chelsea Briggs, a teacher at Marjory Stoneman Douglas in Parkland, said that she "talks to teens every single day and they can't even look her in the eye." She thinks "we need to start coming together and say, "You know what? Let's put the phones down, let's put the computers down, and let's try to figure out where everyone is coming from. We need to stop being on our own agendas and start listening to each other... It has to come to a common ground, there's always a common ground. You show positivity to others, you'll get it right back." One way to accomplish this is to work together on team projects because they get us to talk to each other and work toward a common goal.

JOURNALING BREAK:
Finding a middle ground

- What does cooperation mean to you?
- Write about a time when you had to cooperate with someone. Did it go well? Why or why not?
- Do you like working on projects with a friend? Why or why not?
- Consider how you feel when working within a group toward a common goal – the stress of working with others, time management, busy schedules, different priorities or visions, etc. How were you able to complete the project? How do you think your words and actions made others feel in that scenario?

WE CAN REACH OUT TO DEVELOP RELATIONSHIPS

When we were younger, we made fast friends, whether it was in school or through sports or at camp. As we get older, it gets harder to connect, but we can make an effort to develop relationships by reaching out and taking the first step. Cory Alexander explains that "we must train ourselves to realize that it's not that necessary to have our cell phones glued to our hands and get back to connecting with each other and having conversations with each other. That will develop more empathy and relationships. Relationship is the key to everything."

JOURNALING BREAK:
Reaching out to help

- Write about a time that someone helped you.
  - How did it make you feel?
  - How do you think it made them feel?
- Now, write about a time that you helped another person.
  - Why did you help them?
  - How did it make you feel?
  - How do you think it made them feel?

"When you interact with other cultures and other people, you learn so much, aside from the fact that they cry like you, smile like you, laugh like you."
– Sadiqa Glusman

WE CAN INTERACT WITH PEOPLE FROM DIFFERENT WALKS OF LIFE

Sadiqa Glusman feels strongly that "when you interact with other cultures and other people, you learn so much, aside from the fact that they cry like you, smile like you, laugh like you." We are all more similar than we think, and if we talk to people with an open mind and really listen, then we will understand that.

JOURNALING BREAK:
The human connection

- If you consider that all of us are connected, how should we be treating the Earth?
- How should we be interacting with one another? Why?

CONNECTION PRACTICE:
Common ground

- Go outside, find a comfortable place to sit quietly, and look up at the sky. Realize that it's the same sky that your friends and relatives see, the same stars your grandparents and ancestors could see, and the sun and moon are the same sun and moon that people have been seeing for thousands of years.
- Look at the ground and notice that it's the same ground that friends have walked on, animals have walked on, plants and trees have grown on. The air is shared by other people. The water is used for showering, cleaning, cooking and drinking by people all over the world, all with a common purpose to survive.
- Understand how we are all connected.

WE CAN SPEAK UP AND LISTEN

CASEL's Heather Schwartz says that if "we can make it clear why there's something we need and how we believe it will serve us, then adults will listen." This also goes for our peers too. We can learn to speak and listen with openness and compassion; speak our truths with kindness and without judgment; and be there for each other. There are better ways to resolve disagreements, and mindful communication is at the top of the list.

JOURNALING BREAK:
Resolving conflict with a friend

- Have you ever had a disagreement with a friend while you were working together on a project? How did you resolve it?

- Think of a recent disagreement you had with someone. Write down the words you heard the other person say, and how they could have changed those statements to remove the blame or accusation in them. How would that have helped you to resolve the conflict?
- Do you think mindful communication could have helped you solve it in a better way? If so, how?

WE CAN REALIZE THAT WE ARE NOT ALONE

World Happiness Festival advisor Orlaith O'Sullivan believes that "with practice, we connect to the fact that there are always many joys, and there are always many things going on in the world so that we're connected to others. This is what it means to be a human being." To reiterate a common theme throughout this book, everyone else is feeling some kind of joy, sadness, anger or multiple emotions, just like you, so before you allow yourself to feel isolated or blame others for their demeanors, recognize that you don't know what they are dealing with, and offer up some compassion for yourself and them.

WE CAN COLLABORATE

Simply put, if we can work together, we can find resolutions. It's up to us, our generation, to rise up and stand up for what we believe in. This may be hard because there will always be others who have different beliefs, but if we can share our truths with kindness, then maybe we can do a better job of healing this world and crossing the aisle to get more things accomplished for the betterment of all of us in society.

WE CAN CONNECT WITH KIND PEOPLE

J.G. Larochette says that he "recommends connection for young people by surrounding yourself with compassionate people that care about you and avoiding people who are making you be something you're not." Many of us choose to surround ourselves with people who don't serve us, and by that, I mean people who don't show or reciprocate kindness. We don't have to hold on to toxicity, and we can give ourselves permission to find a group of friends who lifts us up and supports us. Those people don't have to live near us either – the phones are good for something, lol.

WE CAN INSPIRE OTHERS TO WALK THE WALK

If a teen is practicing mindfulness, and a parent or teacher is still screaming or impatient, then it really makes it hard for that teen to be mindful. As my Grandpa George used to say, "It's not our responsibility as parents to raise kids. It's our responsibility to raise adults – kind, compassionate and empathetic adults." But I think we can also teach the adults in a bottom-up approach as well. There's nothing that says that teens can't be the teachers. Let's show them how it's done. After all, Dr. Chris Willard once told me, "The best way to create mindful and compassionate kids and teens is to surround them with compassionate and mindful adults."

JOURNALING BREAK:
Spreading your mindfulness practice

- What are some activities that you do – and that you can share with others – to help center yourself and find a sense of calm?
- How can we best communicate with the adults around us about the hamster wheel of mindfulness?

WE CAN BE MINDFUL, PRESENT AND COMPASSIONATE

Former Congressman Tim Ryan believes that "you have technology and lots of info coming at you that can tend to distract you... and so your mind is not where you are... your mind is in the future and the past. Mindfulness cultivates more awareness, and you'll be aware of what's actually going on inside of you and what people around you are going through, and that leads to compassion." I sometimes have a hard time being present – for example, when I'm having a conversation with my parents at the same time that I'm on my phone. I acknowledge that it's rude and that I should be fully present with them and put the phone down. It's a habit, and like I said throughout this book, no one is perfect, not even me. So, I will continue to do my best to be aware and make a conscious effort to be more present, no matter who I'm with, at any given moment.

JOURNALING BREAK:
Being mindful of others' feelings

Think about these different hypothetical situations, one at a time.

1. You see a student sitting alone in the lunchroom.
2. You learn of a student who is being teased about a speech impediment.
3. You hear a student got into trouble for cheating on a test.

Write about how you think each scenario would make the person feel by considering how you would feel in the same situation. How, if at all, could you help?

EMOTIONAL HYGIENE

If at first you don't succeed, don't quit. Beginning again is a reset, and it's a prime example of gifting yourself with compassion; by affording others the same process, you develop compassion, which leads to empathy, and that's the umbrella under which everything else lies. If you can get to empathy, then you can get to connection, and that leads to inner peace.

Some people call this "cultivating emotional hygiene," which basically means reducing your anxiety, anger, fear, sadness and other challenging emotions. But gaining inner peace doesn't happen overnight. If you can learn how to perform these techniques daily when life isn't particularly stressful, then you'll be able to use these tools when things become overwhelming, traumatic or frustrating... like when none of your technology seems to be working your way, or when you are unexpectedly stuck in the house for months. Cultivating some semblance of inner peace can help when life gets stressful.

13

GETTING TO NEUTRAL

Finding Balance Through Acceptance
and Non-Judgment

When I was younger, I used to think that being mindful and focusing on the now were the same as making a choice to be happy. Now, I understand that it's impossible to be happy 100 percent of the time – and no one expects me to be. Mindfulness helps us to be happier, yes, but life is still life, and we are allowed to feel all of our emotions. Teen life is full of obstacles, and some teens may face traumatic experiences. The goal is to balance the emotions so that we are not overwhelmingly sad or angry all the time. Practicing mindfulness can help us get to neutral, as Grandpa would say, and that's half the battle.

JOURNALING BREAK:
Mindfulness and moods

- When you are feeling down, how do you lift your mood?
- How do you change negative thoughts into positive, or get to a more balanced state?
- What does "getting to neutral" mean to you?

- What are your thoughts or feelings about asking for help? In what situations would you seek someone's advice or counsel?

ACCEPTANCE

Some people believe that the way to get beyond pain, and the manifestation of that pain (whether it be substance abuse, violence, discrimination, etc.), is to first get to a place of acceptance. I'm not sure how I feel about that. Intellectually, I understand it, but as a teen, I can totally understand how this would be really challenging. In fact, I think acceptance is probably considered one of the hardest concepts for teens to grasp and implement. However, I don't think acceptance means that you need to accept life's events as inevitable, unchangeable, excusable or a mark against you as a person. **None of these traumatic events are excusable, none of them are okay.**

I remember seeing a graphic that explained what acceptance is and is not by using the statement, "It's raining." Non-acceptance of rain would be something like, "I wish it wasn't raining. Why does it always have to rain? My day would be better if it was sunny." Acceptance of rain is simply, "Yes, it's raining." It took me a long time to stop grieving after my grandfather passed away because I missed him and wished he was still here in Earth form. What helped me get to a place of acceptance was talking to him about whatever was on my mind, the things I was grateful for, the stuff I wanted to share with him.

JOURNALING BREAK:
Acceptance

- What does "acceptance" mean to you?
  - Do you think it means that we have to accept all of life's events as inevitable, even the traumatic ones?
  - Or does it mean that we should come to a place of acceptance that life, in general, is not perfect, and that we are all human?

Life is imperfect. It can be joyous and exciting, just as it can be scary, stressful and sad. Either way, we need to remind ourselves that these emotions are temporary because everything in life changes, and nothing is stagnant. That's something I've had to accept. If you can have compassion for yourself without judgment as you're experiencing emotions, and remind yourself that emotions change and thoughts come and go, then you can reach acceptance, and maybe even gratitude. For example, "Yes, it's raining, and I am grateful for the rain because it helps food grow," or "Yes, my grandfather is no longer with us in physical form, but I am so grateful for every opportunity I had to be with him and learn from him, and I carry him with me in everything that I do."

One time, I was faced with simultaneous acceptance and gratitude was when I visited a hospital, and the kids, some of whom were bald from treatment and hooked up to tubes, were so happy singing and dancing with Wuf Shanti (of course, I was in the costume feeling sad about their predicaments, but they didn't know that). I looked at their parents standing there watching their kids, and I noticed happiness in their eyes because their children were experiencing joy. But there was also a deep sadness because they knew what their children were going through, and they were uncertain and afraid of the outcome. It was a bittersweet moment for me to find acceptance of these children's hardships, but also gratitude for being able to make them smile.

MANAGING DIFFICULTY

The National Institute of Mental Health defines stress as "the brain and body's response to change, challenge or demand," but there are practices that make it so that stress doesn't affect your health.[37] What do you do with difficult experiences? If you hold on to them, focus on them, or let the blame or anger consume you, then you are going to get stuck on the wrong path. Debra Burdick, the Brain Lady, has an exercise that she teaches called "Changing the Channel," which is basically practicing skills to rewire your brain's negative or unhelpful neuronal pathways to alight more helpful pathways.[38]

ACCEPTANCE PRACTICE:
Rip it up

- Draw something you are upset or mad about, and something positive you can do about it.
- Then, rip up the card to let go of the anger...
- ... And don't forget about the positive solution you wrote down! Instead, do it so you can resolve and accept the situation.

We can make a different choice: to focus on gratitude, thereby moving beyond any potential self-harming behaviors. In order to get to a place of self-awareness, self-love and inner peace, maybe we need to first come to accept that we are not perfect – no one is, nor is life perfect. But if we can become self-aware of our self-critical thoughts, then we can move past them, manage our difficult feelings before they escalate and allow self-compassion into our lives. I like to think of it this way: If we can love ourselves as much as we love our pets, see ourselves as our pets see us, and accept that we are worthy of such love, then we can have better relationships with ourselves, and know that we are enough and that it's okay to be exactly who we are. (Our dogs really do love us that much.)

> **"'Without judgment' is the key, because instead of criticizing the thoughts, it's like, 'Oh, thoughts.' And that's the biggest gift."**
>
> **– J.G. Larochette**

NON-JUDGMENT

This is where non-judgment comes in. The words "without judgment" are in the definition of mindfulness because, if you can recognize your thoughts without judgment, then you can let them go more easily. As J.G. Larochette said, "'Without judgment' is the key, because instead of criticizing the thoughts, it's like, 'Oh, thoughts.' And that's the biggest gift. So many of us are caught in wanting to be perfect, instead of just BEing. We have to stop perfection messaging because we are overwhelming our nervous systems. We are not our thoughts, and we are not our emotions. Experiences of the mind come and go like clouds, and as long as we don't jump on them and get carried away into an untrue reality, then we can see what is truly real."

We need to learn to be less judgmental of ourselves and accept ourselves for who we are, our strengths and weakness. Amy Burke said, "Young people should learn to listen to their inner voices more and trust themselves. It's a form of self-care, and making yourself a priority is really important." You can't stop judging others or accept others until you first stop judging yourself, and that can be easier said than done – but it is doable. Like everything else, it just takes practice, patience and self-compassion. When distracting thoughts enter your mind, you can acknowledge them and release them without judgment, knowing that those thoughts do not control or define you. You can replace them with a positive thought as well.

JOURNALING BREAK:
Letting go of judgment

- Write about a time that you judged yourself or another person unfairly.
- Then, write about a time that you gave yourself a break or accepted another person as they were.
- Be sure to write about how you felt after judging versus being non-judgmental.

A friend of mine, Taylor, shared that she and her best friend had started drifting apart, and it was hard to accept that the person she'd always go to was no longer there. She felt her friend was often focusing on the negative, and it was making Taylor feel more negative, which she didn't like. Ultimately, she had to take a step back from the friendship, and that hurt, but she had to accept the option that was right for her.

Taylor went on to explain that she also had to learn to love herself more and shut out the pressure on social media to look a certain way because it got to her head and

GETTING TO NEUTRAL

made her doubt her self-worth. She advises that one way to address that self-perceived judgment is by taking time off social media and focusing on improving yourself for you, not for others. Her advice would be to keep a positive mindset, take a step back, take a break and regroup, look at your life, and remind yourself of all the things you have to be grateful for. To help center herself, she usually breathes in and out, counts backward from 100 or makes more of an effort to reach out and connect with others.

FORGIVENESS PRACTICE:
Directing love and kindness

Let's try a heartfelt practice and direct love and kindness to another person. Usually, we do this with people we love already – it's much harder to do it for someone that you are not happy with in a given moment – but it teaches us about acceptance, forgiveness and compassion.

- Minimize distractions around you and sit in a comfortable position.
- Close your eyes if you feel comfortable, or focus on a spot on the floor. Notice what your body connects with.
- Let your breath become smooth, breathing in love and compassion on the inhale, and breathing out whatever you need to release, alongside love and compassion, on the exhale.
- While you are doing this, visualize someone that you are feeling annoyed with or having a conflict with.

- Now, visualize them surrounded by light and think about how you are grateful for their health, safety and happiness.
- Repeat the mantra, "I am grateful for your health, safety and happiness."
- Continue doing this for five breath cycles – a breath in and out is one cycle.
- Notice how you feel after sending these warm wishes to that person. Take and release a compassionate breath for yourself as well. When you are ready, gently open your eyes.

JOURNALING BREAK:
Forgiveness

- Reflect and write about a time you forgave yourself or someone else, and how it made you feel.

Teenagers have a tendency to judge not only others, but especially themselves – harshly. Learning to be less insecure and self-critical and releasing self-judgment are key components of living a grounded life in the here and now. We are each unique; we are each special; we are each worthy. The more you consciously practice this, the fewer negative thoughts you will have, and you can give yourself a pat on the back for any progress, even if it's one less negative thought. It's totally expected to have these thoughts, and when they occur, you can simply watch as they float away and disappear, and then you can begin again.

RELEASING PRACTICE:
Letting go of emotions

- Find a comfortable sitting position, and in silence, notice how you are feeling.
- Give attention to where you are holding the emotion in your body, and with every exhale of your breath, have the deliberate and conscious intention to release tension from that body part, as well as to release the emotion so that you are no longer holding on to it, no longer allowing it any power over you.
- Focus on seeing that emotion leave your body and letting it go by saying goodbye to it, to whatever doesn't serve you.
- Visualize yourself laying on the ground and looking up at the peaceful sky, feeling the calm.
- If thoughts and emotions enter your brain, that's okay – watch as they float away on the clouds and disappear.

RELEASING PRACTICE:
Surfing the waves

The above exercise can also be done with waves.
- Each wave is an emotion that comes and goes.
- Watch as you expertly surf the waves.
- Now, watch as the thoughts disappear one by one. Feel the tension start to ease out of your body. Notice your breathing.

JOURNALING BREAK:
Handling stress and pressure

Consider the situations below and write about how you would handle them.

1. You are upset because your parents want you to stop talking to your friends on the phone and go to sleep.
2. You are jealous because your friend seems to be doing better in a sport than you, or getting better grades, or is spending more time with another friend than you.
3. You are sad and worried because your family pet is sick and at the veterinarian, or a close relative/friend is in the hospital.
4. You are not doing well on the SAT practice exams and you're feeling the pressure big time.

Dave Smith said, "We live in hard times right now. There's a lot of uncertainty and scary things going on. But there are also a lot of beautiful things going on. Focus on yourself and what's most meaningful to you because that's where genuine happiness comes from." So, ask yourself, can you be genuinely happy without gratitude? My opinion is that, at the very least, gratitude must come first because it helps you get to neutral and feel some inner peace and contentment with your life. Better yet, gratitude leads to happiness – more on that in the next chapter.

14

GRATITUDE

Developing an Attitude of Gratitude – and Expressing It

People traditionally talk about gratitude most during Thanksgiving. Yes, Thanksgiving is the designated official holiday for being grateful (at least it is in the US), but we should be expressing gratitude every day, right?

It's important to teach all about positivity, kindness and gratitude because it's a building block to everything else. One of our main messages at Wuf Shanti is "smile and say thank you," and we call it our gratitude mantra. A mentor of mine, Erika Lee, told me that she describes gratitude to kids as finding the coolest pair of "miracle glasses" and putting them on. Erika explains that the glasses are perfect: They're free, they fit your eyes perfectly, they're really light on the face, and they're super easy to find. Most importantly, though, you just have to wake up in the morning, put them on and choose to see everything through the lenses as miracles, just as the glasses' name suggests.

I guess for this book, a good question to ask would be, "Are teens grateful?" And if so, "What are teens actually grateful for?" And taking it a step further, "Can they learn to be?"

I think we are naturally thankful for the food we eat, the water we drink, and our families and friends. But can we go beyond that? What about in difficult times? Can we practice gratitude authentically?

> One of my friends, Stephen, said that consciously practicing gratitude helped save his life because it reminded him that there are good things to focus on, and stuff could always be worse.

AN ATTITUDE OF GRATITUDE

Moving from a state of mind of entitlement for what we are given to a mindset of gratitude and appreciation is hard for a teen these days, but it's not impossible. For every yin, there is a yang; for every negative, there is a positive; and you have a choice of what you focus on. An attitude of gratitude can turn someone's life around in a profound way. Being thankful for what you have – instead of focusing on what you don't have – and putting positivity into the universe will ultimately attract positivity and gratitude to you, because what you give out, you get back. My Grandpa Alan's favorite song was "Always Look on the Bright Side of Life," from the Monty Python musical *Spamalot*, and he sang that song even when he was at the end of his life. I think of him singing that song, and it helps me to focus on the fun things, like the fact that we got to see Frankie Valli in concert and lots of Broadway shows together, and that he traveled with me and was front and center when I delivered my TEDx Talk.

During the Covid-19 pandemic, it may have been hard for some teens to find gratitude. I really had to meditate on this one too, and here's a perspective that I came up with: If life was normal, and I had more distractions, then I wouldn't have had the time to focus on school, and I may not have gotten straight As. If I'd had places to go and people to see, then I wouldn't have been able to be so creative and start multiple passion projects, which made my time at home worth it. Also, how many teens actually spent that much time with their families pre-pandemic? And for me, that was a good thing (as much as they do annoy me sometimes, which I think is customary). As an adult, I know I will look back in gratitude for the amount of time I got to spend with my family before leaving for college.

JOURNALING BREAK:
Gratitude

- Why is it important for us to recognize and express gratitude? What do you think that can do for us? What do you think we gain from focusing on things that we are grateful for?
- Fold a piece of paper vertically into thirds, or draw two lines down, making three columns. Write something that's upsetting you on the left side of the paper, something that could have been worse in the middle, and something that is better or can make it better on the right side.
- Complete three of these gratitude prompts:
  - I am grateful for these three things I see…
  - I am grateful for these three things I hear…
  - I am grateful for these three things that are yellow…
  - I am grateful for these three people in my family…
  - I am grateful for these three animals…
  - I am grateful for these three activities…
- Make a list of ten things you are grateful for. Go beyond identifying who or what you are grateful for and focus on why you are grateful. Here are some prompts to help you get started:
  - I am grateful for my friend because…
  - I am grateful for my pet because…

- ○ I am grateful for my family because...
- ○ Something amazing happened today, and I am grateful for it because...
- ○ I am grateful for who I am because...

GRATITUDE FOR THOSE WHO'VE MADE AN IMPACT IN YOUR LIFE

I once saw a post by Dr. Chris Willard that asked the following question: "Who is no longer in your life that you are still grateful to have known?"[39] I really liked that question because it made me stop and think; it also really made me think about my gratitude practice. I had a really good friend for many years, and we did everything together – we practically grew up in each others' houses. We are still connected on socials, but we no longer talk. We now have new groups of friends. But here's the thing: I am still grateful for that person because they gave me one of my first lessons in friendship. And I've come to realize that no matter what paths our lives take, we will always be connected. For example, this friend still reaches out on my birthday and reached out when my grandfather died, and I very much appreciated that. I would do the same thing in return if I learned of an event like that happening to them. And of course, I only wish good things for my old friend. The question Dr. Willard posted made me think about the meaning and lessons of friendship. Ask yourself: Who are you grateful for that is no longer in your life?

If you are very lucky, then you have someone in both your personal life and in your school life for whom you can express gratitude. For me, in my school life, I'm grateful for my guidance counselors, Mrs. Dominguez, Mrs. Lily, Mr. Ziccardi and Mrs. Siwek. They care about their students beyond the matters at hand. Everyone reading this book has probably had an issue that they needed to discuss with a guidance counselor, and maybe you thought you could only talk to them about school stuff; however, you can talk to them about whatever is going on in your life.

When people ask me what to do if they are facing difficult times or feeling sad, upset or stressed, I always suggest talking. And that means to anyone you feel comfortable with – just don't hold it in. Talk to a friend or a trusted adult: a parent, teacher, coach, mentor, etc. Just talk. Sometimes, my generation seems to forget how to do this, but hopefully, you have someone in your life who reminds you. I can go talk to my guidance counselors whenever I need to, and I know that they listen and care, and that they will help if they can. We are different people (male, female, Black, white, older and younger, working and in school), and yet we care a lot about each other. I know they'll advocate for my best interests.

If you have a guidance counselor or teacher who has been there for you, do something nice for them, like write a thank-you note to let them know they have made a difference in your life. If you haven't met your guidance counselor yet, go introduce yourself – you may meet someone who becomes a huge source of support. Our emotions aren't going away, so it's good to have someone to talk to because the way around it is through it.

"THINK WELL TO BE WELL"

It is possible for all of us to cultivate inner strength, compassion and gratitude by learning to cope with challenging emotions in a non-destructive way, a way that honors us and those around us. Just as kindness and laughter are contagious, so too is gratitude. Ever notice that little kids laugh a lot and, when they're upset, they usually get over it and let it go really quickly? That's because they focus on the positive, a form of gratitude. Haris Lender of Kidding Around Yoga says that "Laughter is the best medicine. We teach kids when they are young that we can heal ourselves with positivity and laughter."

At Wuf Shanti, we tell younger kids to make up a fake laugh, and then we ask their friend or sibling to copy their laugh. Then, the copier gets to make up one of their own for their partner to mimic. We have them keep doing that until the laughter becomes authentic (trust me, it always does because it's catchy). And then we explain that our brains don't know we're pretending. Even as a teenager, I can do a variation on that. When I'm feeling upset, sometimes I like to deliberately make myself smile.

Great-Grandpa Jack once told me a story about helping a woman find her lost car in a mall parking lot (in the days before iPhones and car alarms). She was super upset, crying, and had been walking in circles for an hour in the hot sun. Grandpa wanted to cheer her up, so he said something funny that would make her laugh. He said he would help her find her car, and then he said, "Oh, by the way, you may want to walk backward while we look for your car." She asked why. And he answered, "To get the other side of your face sunburned to match this side!"

Well, maybe it was the stress of the situation, but once he made her laugh, she couldn't stop laughing, and then they caused a scene because everyone around them stopped to see what was happening, and then THEY all started laughing... *for no reason...* and everyone was all laughing together – and they didn't even know why! Grandpa knew then what scientists have since proven: that smiling is catchy... and healing.

It may sound weird, but your brain doesn't know that you're not really happy if you're laughing or smiling. It simply gets the signal from your body that you're smiling, and then it thinks you're happy. When I've tried it, it makes me feel better, at least enough to begin a mindfulness practice and achieve inner calm in that moment. When we have compassion for ourselves, we have compassion for others. The same magic happens with gratitude. And we're back to the chain reaction!

My Grandma Nola does something similar with dancing because she says dancing helps her feel better and celebrate life. It's like a mind-body connection, and I definitely believe that our minds can affect our bodies and vice versa. As my Great-Grandpa Jack used to say, "Think well to be well," and even though it may be difficult sometimes, that's what I strive to do in my practice.

Most of the time, his mantra holds true, and I agree that positive thoughts can help us to feel happier and healthier. But now, because of my Grandpa Alan, I also believe that when hard or traumatic things happen and we can't get to a happy place, that's okay – we may still be able to get to neutral. Todd Wolfenberg pointed out, "Nothing is permanent. Throughout the day, you'll have changes. You'll feel good for part of the day, bad for part of the day, and that's expected. If you have these mindful tools to use when you're not feeling as strong as you want to be, they can help you go to your next event with a clear space and not bring the negativity with you."

GRATITUDE PRACTICE:
Threes

One positivity and gratitude practice we like to teach at Wuf Shanti is focusing on three things that you are thankful for each day, the good things in your life, either in the morning to start the day, or in the evening before bedtime.

- These can be simple things, like something that made you smile that day, a funny TV show, a bird chirping, a butterfly flying around or playing with your dog.
- Or they can be things you're thankful for, like your health, the sunshine, family, friends, the book you're reading, the test you did okay on – anything you want.

Doing a daily gratitude practice is worthwhile because it's kind of like you're exercising your brain and building up the muscles that you need, so when you're *really* stressed, you'll already know how to implement these tools to help yourself.

When you practice gratitude, especially in difficult times, it helps you focus on the positive and remember that there are some good things in the world, bringing you one step closer to feeling happier again. J.G. Larochette once told me, "I always like to start my morning with a daily practice of gratitude. That helps me be present, so I don't automatically start thinking about negative thoughts or what I have to do that day. One of the most harmful messages that we often believe is that love, happiness, joy, peace [and] gratitude are things that we have to attain through the external world and not from within. We often go down the external path looking for all these and suffer greatly because of it. Once we realize that the most important path to experience these is cultivating them deeply inward, we can then realize what we have been searching for has always been there."

SEIZE THE DAY

Every morning is a new day, and we can choose to be positive. I remember once when I was younger and upset about something, my Great-Grandpa Jack would make me smile by singing a song with me called "Enjoy Yourself While You're Still in the Pink." I recently saw the video again, and it put a big smile on my face. His lesson, as usual, was about thinking well and having gratitude for every day. If a day is hard, remind yourself that you had happy or peaceful moments, and each of those moments in time is special, so you should remember them and be grateful for them. Practicing this daily helps us develop a positive attitude that allows us to appreciate the little moments that life offers.

> **"Give a title to the chapters of your life, and project into the future. What's your vision?"**
> **– Matt Dewar**

Matt Dewar said something to me that really stuck with me. He said, "The average person lives a lifespan of 30,000 days. Give a title to the chapters of your life, and project into the future. What's your vision? Imagine a jar filled with 30,000 pebbles, and this morning when you woke up, you pulled a pebble out of the jar of your life that you'll never put back in there. You have a pebble of your life in your hand, so what are you going to do with it? When the day is over, that pebble is gone. It's so important to value your most precious resource, which is not renewable, and that's time." If we can remember that every day is one less pebble in the jar of life, then we can find something to be grateful for in the present moment. Appreciate the good.

GRATITUDE PRACTICE:
Visualizing gratitude

- Choose something that makes you feel happy or lifts you up, something you can do to take care of your mental state, something that makes you smile.

- Now, close your eyes if you are comfortable doing so and envision your negative thoughts as clouds. Watch them float away.
- Take one thing from the list that makes you happy and pretend to hold it to your heart.
- Take deep breaths in and out as you visualize this happiness filling you up and surrounding you like beautiful light. (The visualized light can be any color, rainbow, sunshine, etc. – whatever you prefer.)
- Know that no one can take that feeling away from you. The power is within you.

15

INTENTION

Making the World a Better Place by Using Your Voice

Positive chain reactions can heal the world. Dr. Dan Siegel told me that there's "incredible possibility for what adolescents can do to create a healthier, more connected, more compassionate, more integrated world. Adolescents will be the leaders of directing change on this planet, and [...] we can tap into the potential and creativity of adolescents to really solve some of the world's greatest challenges."

It is possible to re-wire your brain, overcome the negativity bias and find your true intention with a little practice and a little patience. Stress and pain are part of life, and the only thing you can control is how you respond to it. Dan Harris believes that having a purpose helps you stay mentally healthy. He said, "For teens, staying engaged in a healthy way, given all the other responsibilities teens have... is the way to not feel like you got run over by a truck all the time because you're doing something positive, no matter how small." We can all learn to live in the moment and appreciate what is happening now. Once you are on the path to healing, you can find your purpose and use your voice to make sure that others don't have the same experiences that you did and/or make the world a little brighter. That's what being an advocate is all about!

JOURNALING BREAK:
Intention

Consider your purpose in life.
- How can you make this world better?
- Outline an action plan to make that happen.

DO YOUR PART

Teen Jordan Temeres said that his "number one answer to making the world a better place is spreading awareness." We (teens) are our future. We are the ones that have the opportunity to jump off the hamster wheel and make positive change. As Jennifer Miller said, "The magic of the teen world is figuring out how you can contribute to the world and what you can do that can make a difference and what your purpose is. How are you going to contribute to the world, and how can you start today, in any small way? How can you make a difference at home, at school, in the community?" By learning to form new positive intentions, you can manifest what you want your world to be like. This does not mean that bad things will never happen to you or that you will never face challenges, but rather that you will know how to cope with those things in a healthier way, which will allow you to live a more peaceful, loving and happier existence. Todd Wolfenberg thinks teens should "learn to tap into both opportunities and challenges because they can channel that in a positive direction and change the world, and that's really powerful."

As far back as I can remember, probably starting when I was five years old, my mom would make me learn about charities and how to give back to help people. It seemed natural to me to become a peer counselor in school, as well as to take my great-grandfather's teachings and pay it forward by teaching others about mindfulness. Nobody ever told me I couldn't accomplish whatever I wanted. I really think that if we believe in something, then we have to be vocal and make ourselves heard. We have to use our voices and make this world a better place to live in.

As Dr. Sam Himmelstein said, "Teens have the key to the magic to help create real change on this planet in many different ways, and I want to encourage you to hold on to that and do whatever you need to do to keep being you and keep finding yourself and what drives you and makes you feel purposeful on the planet." One good example of advocacy comes from American Idol contestant Taylor Fagins, who wrote a song about the killing of Black people. Taylor isn't a teen, but he is a young adult, and I wanted to include this as an example of using our passions and talents, while at the same time making an impact on the world. The lyrics are powerful, and Taylor found a creative way to make people listen. Another well-known advocate is Greta Thunberg, who started taking the helm of environmental activism on behalf of our generation and future generations when she was only 15. There are many other awesome teen advocates, thankfully, and I'm grateful to all of them. If we don't do it, then who will? The world needs us now more than ever.

JOURNALING BREAK:
Making your mark

- What do you want out of life?
- What do you hope to accomplish?
- How do you want to make your mark? Why?
- Write about your greatest wish for your future. How you will go about making that a reality, with integrity?

FIND YOUR PURPOSE

Mindfulness-based social-emotional learning (MBSEL) techniques help me deal with stress, but having a purpose – something positive to focus on – has helped me too. Pursuing my purpose – to be mindful and encourage others to do the same – hasn't all been fun and games. For one thing, there are some misconceptions about mindfulness. Some school leaders think these mindful practices are a religion, but they're not. They're totally secular and for everyone. If someone tries to tell me that mindfulness is a religion, I usually say something like, "Sure, if your religion is peace, love and kindness."

Sometimes teens give me excuses as to why they can't be mindful, like they don't have time, or they don't want to sit cross-legged with their eyes closed and their hands in a mudra position (another misconception), or they feel embarrassed. To achieve my purpose, I have to overcome all of those excuses by calmly explaining the benefits of mindfulness, and showing how it can be practiced by anyone, anywhere, in any way. In reading this book, you've already learned that mindfulness can be practiced standing up, walking around, playing a sport, drawing, singing a song, in the morning, at night, for one minute, ten minutes, alone or with others. There's no "one right way" to do it, and the goal is not to be perfect, but to develop focus and compassion, and take time for yourself to find balance.

> **"The purpose of sitting down is to rise up."**
> **– Shelly Tygielsky**

If you're wondering what mindfulness has to do with purpose, I heard a great explanation from author and mindfulness expert Shelly Tygielsky. She said, "The purpose of sitting down is to rise up." For example, I believe that everyone, in all communities, should have access to MBSEL education, and that's what I will be working on in the coming years. I do it not only to create positive change and make an impact on the world, but also because it makes me feel happier to do it. Whitney Stewart said there's "great research to show that the more you do for others, the more happiness you feel."

JOURNALING BREAK:
Finding your purpose

- What do you think are the biggest problems in our society, and how should we address them?
- Make a list of positive ways you can impact the world.

CHASE YOUR PASSIONS

Now (in the editing phase of this book), I go to Syracuse University and study at the Newhouse School, where I am majoring in broadcast and digital journalism, and also minoring in sports management and psychology/mindfulness. Why? Because my passions are sports and mental health. If a broadcast career can lead me to talking with athletes about their mental health and end the stigma, then I can help future generations.

Find something you're passionate about and know that you can be an agent of change simply by using your voice, and it will make you feel good too. Discuss your ideas with parents, friends, teachers or anyone who supports you. No matter how they react, remember this: If you believe in a cause, and you want to do something about it, then make yourself an expert in it and do it. As my Grandpa Alan used to say: Power abhors a vacuum. Simply put, don't wait for someone else, don't wait to be asked. Just do it. If you see a void, fill it. Seize the opportunity, assume the responsibility. If you stand around waiting for the call, it may never come.

While you should be respectful of everyone, you should also feel free to always voice your opinions and not feel obligated to keep quiet and deferential. Our generation, with fresh points of view, are critical to the healing of the world. As teen Emanuelle Sippy put it, "Teens should know they actually do have the power to do something about whatever is bothering them and make changes. Recognize you have the capacity to change something."

JOURNALING BREAK:
Reaching the finish line

- Write about a great accomplishment, how it made you feel, and whether it changed the way you think about or tackle situations that arise in life.
- What does being a leader mean to you?

I'm not a politician so I can't change the law. But I can do everything in my power to make sure that mental health issues, violence and self-harm stop becoming the norm by reaching the next generation and teaching them how to deal with their emotions. Similarly, Amy Eva had a message for teens: "We're good enough the way we are. There's no need to compare yourself to other people. You have a unique role and purpose in this world and something to give to all of us, a purpose beyond yourself. We need your voice and need to hear from teens and need you to contribute to the greater good."

You can help too. We all have our strengths. Find yours and make this world better. Regardless of your political beliefs, be like my grandpa and become friends with someone across the aisle. Talk to a stranger, extend a hand, help someone else today. People appreciate small acts of kindness. Send them an article to let them know you're thinking about them. Help others succeed. Be a source of support for others. That way, as my grandpa taught me, it vastly increases the chance that they'll be there for you when you need it.

And don't forget to be a source of love, too. As Joe Lockett said beautifully, "Once you get a platform, you have to show the generation coming up behind you that you care. Give back to your community starting early. Leave a blueprint, leave the door open, for the next generation." Teach teens to do the same. The time is now. As Argos Gonzalez so aptly put it, "Teens can do a much better job than we did. They will meet all the challenges they are facing and not only survive them, but thrive. Teens your age are the most prepared, smartest, savvy generation, the generation this world needs."

JOURNALING BREAK:
A final message

- If you could share one message with teens, what would it be?
- If you could share one message with adults (your parents, teachers or even random strangers), what would it be?

16

A GUIDE ON YOUR ROAD TO SUCCESS

Your Quick Reference After Reading

You've reached the end of the book, and you've covered a lot of ground. Thank you so much for taking the time to read through it. I want this book to be a reference for you, but I also know you can't read it from front to back every time you need mindfulness guidance. So, I've added a final chapter with every teen's favorite resource: a cheat sheet!

The number one thing you need to do to get on the path to a successful, mindful life is to just start. I don't want to sound like a broken record, but make an effort to communicate and connect with others, be kind to yourself and to others, and above all, believe in yourself. You are special and worthy, so don't let anyone tell you otherwise.

JOURNALING BREAK:
A mindful check-in

Choose and answer two of these prompts:
- What would make you happy right now?
- What is going right in your life?
- What is the nicest thing someone has said to you, and how did it make you feel?

- When did you experience joy this week?
- What do you love about yourself?
- What are you really proud of having accomplished?
- Who means the world to you, and why?
- What is something nice that a friend did for you, and how did it make you feel?
- What inspires you the most?
- What do you like about the way you look/act?
- Will you choose happy or sad? Positive or negative?
- What are some positive ways that you can manage stress, anger and anxiety?
- How can you best get to neutral?

I started on this journey years ago when my great-grandfather passed away, and I wanted to pay his teachings forward. It was my Great-Grandpa Jack's mantra, "Think well to be well," that started Wuf Shanti. As I grew up, so did Wuf Shanti, and thanks to my Grandpa Alan, my views on mindfulness have evolved.

My definition of mindfulness is being focused on the now, without judgment and with kindness to ourselves and others. When we can cope with our emotions and stress, and not worry about yesterday or tomorrow, then we can be happier and healthier. There are so many different ways to practice. You don't have to sit a certain way with your eyes closed, and it's not about being 100 percent happy. Grandpa Alan taught me that, yes, we want to learn to be more positive and get to a happier place, but sometimes getting to neutral is okay too.

Find a practice that resonates with you, and do it for five minutes every day, even if you're in a good headspace at the moment. That way, when stressful things happen, you'll already know how to deal with them in a healthy way, and you'll be better able to navigate the ups and downs of life. We don't wake up one morning knowing how to be mindful. It's something we need to train our brains to do, just as we work out to build our muscles. We each have about 50,000 random thoughts going through our heads every day, and that's normal. We need to be able to be aware of those thoughts and feelings, acknowledge them without judgment and let them go.

Something that I especially like to tell teens is that no one even has to know you're doing a mindful practice. It can be done anywhere, at any time – even something as simple as taking some deep breaths or listening to your favorite song may resonate with you.

Over 6,000 scientific studies have shown that mindfulness helps reduce anxiety and depression, lower blood pressure and increase focus, and it helps you get better grades and form better relationships, along with a ton of other mental and physical benefits.[40] You don't have to take my word for it – just give it a try for a few weeks and see how it makes you feel. Remember that every minute is a new opportunity to begin again. If you're practicing and a random thought comes into your mind, that's okay – release it and begin again.

Stress is a pretty standard thing to feel, something every single person on this planet deals with at one point or another, and that's why social-emotional learning (SEL) is so vital to teach. I believe that mindfulness-based social-emotional learning (MBSEL) and emotional intelligence (EI) should be part of the core curriculum in schools. Knowing these mindful techniques can help us in a big way. Everyone experiences strong emotions. We all feel anxious, sad or upset sometimes, and it's okay to feel those emotions; the trick is becoming aware of them and knowing how to deal with them in a healthy way. It's not about never feeling sad or upset or anxious; it's about allowing yourself to have those emotions and knowing how to process them productively.

Learning these techniques can help us respond instead of reacting and pause before we speak. By taking a second to observe what's happening right now in the present moment, we are better able to proceed with awareness and kindness, and this will help us to resolve potential conflict in a healthy way, with better and kinder communication, which can strengthen our relationships.

Self-care is really important too, especially for people who are hard on themselves a lot, really busy or always helping others. We tend to forget to take time for ourselves. For example, I often have to remind myself to put my phone down so that I can connect with others more, maybe go play golf or basketball or go to bed at a reasonable hour. These are all things that will help my mental health if I do them on a daily basis, and I think they'll help you, too.

We also need to think of others. Random acts of kindness are so easy to do, and they go a very long way. Not only do you make someone else feel good, but you will feel good as well. Kindness is catchy, and it will come back to you. You will notice that you feel more gratitude too.

Other people are dealing with their own stresses and life experiences, and they may be having a difficult time dealing with their emotions too. Always remember that you're not alone. Try to find that one person you can talk to, the one cause you are passionate about that gives you a purpose, and/or that one mindful technique that helps you. Make sure that you take care of yourself because you are important.

When we hit tough times, this is when mindfulness comes into play. If we've been practicing it all along, then we have the tools to help with stressful situations. Being mindful helps us in processing our emotions and remaining calm. We can use the techniques we've learned to be aware of and name our emotions, without judgment, and then we can let them go. It's totally okay to be anxious – I am too, it's normal. But we all need to remind ourselves to take time out for ourselves every day and be present in the moment. Do your breathing techniques, partake in mindful movement and yoga, practice meditation, repeat affirmations, engage in positive thinking or perform whatever healthy coping mechanism helps you handle stress and anxiety. Do what you can to control your environment and try to bring your mind back from the past or future. Focus on now, and while you're at it, send some love out into the universe. If there was ever a time for mindfulness, now is that time.

I'm so grateful for every single experience I've had, for all that I've learned, for every mentor who has provided guidance, for all the people I've met, for every expert I've had the honor to speak with, and for every child or teen we've been able to help in any way. It's hasn't always been easy, but even through the tough times, I've learned so many great lessons about myself, who I want to be as a human being, how I want to contribute to the world and how to connect with people. And I'm still learning every day. These tools have helped me so much in my daily life to deal with stress and cope with emotions, and I'm glad I can share them with others.

All I know for sure is that change is constant. MBSEL is helpful to us in coping with the strong emotions and daily stress that we will all inevitably face throughout our lives, but there's no one-size-fits-all mindfulness technique. With that in mind, go back through this book and try some of the different mindful practices we include for teens and answer (or re-answer) some self-reflection journal questions as well. Find the ones that resonate with you.

I truly hope this book has helped you in some way. I believe that our minds can control our bodies, and if we all try to lead lives of wellness, empathy and compassion, then we can make this world a better place. Success and happiness are intricately connected, and we can learn how to let go of resentment and anger and how to cope in healthy ways. If we want to be successful, then we can start with consciously choosing gratitude and inner calm, and being generous and kind to ourselves and others. It will come back to us. It's all about health and wellness, peace and positivity. Attaining a mindful life of inner peace is achievable if we work toward it.

So, you may have started this book wondering, "*Why should I spend my time reading this book?*"

Hopefully, I've answered that question for you.

Wishing you health and happier-ness always on your journey to get to neutral. Onward.

ABOUT THE AUTHOR

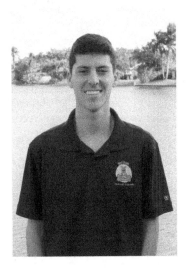

Teen mental health education advocate Adam Avin created the Wuf Shanti Children's Wellness Foundation, a 501c3 non-profit organization, to teach mindfulness and social-emotional learning, so children 3–17 years old can live in health and wellness, and peace and positivity. Adam also founded the Kids' Association for Mindfulness in Education, and the international online Mindful Kids Peace Summit.

Adam is certified in Mindfulness-Based Stress Reduction for Teens, Kidding Around Yoga and the Emotion Code, and is the youngest meditation instructor at Yoga International, Inner Explorer and Stressed Teens. He also has been in publications such as *Mindful* magazine, *Psychology Today*, the Tiger Woods Foundation's magazine, *goop* magazine, the CASEL newsletter, LA Yoga, *Chicken Soup for the Soul: Think Positive Live Happy*, and many others.

Adam gave a TEDxYouth@KC Talk about getting mindful and social-emotional learning programs into our education system, why mental health education is so important to stopping violence, and how we can use our voices to make a positive difference in the world. He also was honored to be the Keynote Speaker for the Broward Mental Health Summit and to have served as a part of the inaugural fellowship for the Kevin Love Fund, a non-profit organization that focuses on getting mental health curriculum into schools.

Adam is a Posse Scholar for the Syracuse University Newhouse School Class of 2026. He will be majoring in broadcast and digital journalism and minoring in either psychology/mindfulness and contemplative studies.

For more information, please visit the Wuf Shanti online:
- https://wufshanti.com/
- https://www.facebook.com/wufshanti/
- https://www.linkedin.com/company/wufshanti/

ACKNOWLEDGMENTS

There are so many people to thank who have helped me along this journey.

I owe a lot of what is now Wuf Shanti Children's Wellness Foundation to my Great-Grandpa Jack, who taught me the main mantra that started it all, "Think well to be well"; to my Grandpa Alan, who taught me to "look on the bright side," "get to neutral," and "never quit"; and to my mom Marni Becker-Avin, who is the absolute best organizer, cheerleader, business manager and editor. She has worked so hard to help me, and I could not have done any of this without her guidance and support.

Some other amazing people who have significantly influenced my life include my Great-Grandma Lorraine, Grandma Nola, Saba Shaul, Grandma Debbie, Aunt Mor, Aunt Ilana, my little sister Sabrina, and of course, my dad Roie Avin (who not only helps compose the Wuf Shanti music, but who has also been in charge of the website, the PR and the social media, not to mention that I get my love of sports, podcasting and music from him). I love each of these people so much and am so grateful for their daily presence in my life. And to those who watch over me, including my Great-Grandma Rita, Safta Shula and Grandpa George, I hope you are all proud of me.

I also want to acknowledge Erika Lee for letting me sit in on her yoga instructions with mom and believing in Wuf Shanti from the very beginning; and my Aunt Gail, who was my first art teacher and helped me learn to draw the original Wuf Shanti.

I've been lucky enough to have some great mentors as well, including Helen Maffini of MindBE Education, who helped me start the Mindful Kids Peace Summit; Dr. Amy Salzman of

Still Quiet Mind, who helped me start the Kids Association for Mindfulness in Education; Gina Biegel of Stressed Teens, who allowed me to be the only teen ever certified in MBSR-T; Bob Roth of the David Lynch Foundation, who helped me with my TEDx; Dr. Bradley Nelson of Discover Healing, who allowed me to be the only teen certified in the Emotion Code; and Laura Bakosh of Inner Explorer, who invited me to be a meditation instructor on the IE platform.

Our Board of Advisors on the Wuf Shanti Children's Wellness Foundation is compromised of pediatricians, psychologists, yoga practitioners, meditation practitioners, mindfulness practitioners, non-profit organizations, educators, media consultants, authors and more. These wonderful humans have been supportive from day one, and I thank each of you as well: Laura Bakosh, Gina Biegel, Amy Burke, Ruthi Davis, Amy Eva, Rachel Friedland, Sadiqa Glusman, Argos Gonzalez, Adam Harrison, Kevin Hawkins, Harry Jho, Dr. Robin Leader-Landau, Haris Lender, Helen Maffini, Brad Meltzer, Jennifer Miller, Dr. Bradley Nelson, Maureik Robison, Bob Roth, Supna Shah, Dr. Lisa Sirota-Weiner, Dave Smith, Perry Sofferman, Terri Cooper-Space, Kim Tegeler, Donnie Vick, Rita Weisskoff and Dr. Christopher Willard.

Wuf Shanti has been on many platforms, and I want to thank them for believing in our content: Common Sense Media Network (safe-streaming for kids); SF PBS (South Florida Public Broadcasting Stations); KidoodleTV (safe-streaming service for kids); Adventure to Learning (health and fitness programming in schools); the Children's Television Network (the positive programming station in children's hospitals across the globe); and Yoga International (who invited me to be their youngest meditation instructor for teens). Along those lines, I want to thank everyone at the Broward Mental Health Summit and TEDx@KC for inviting me to speak (which, I'm not going to lie, was frightening, even for a mindful teen like me). The TEDx especially was an amazing experience that I will never forget and will always treasure because it was the last trip that my Grandpa Alan and I took together.

There are some organizations that have been amazing, consistent collaborators, and I am grateful for them as well: Kidding Around Yoga, Stressed Teens, Inner Explorer, WeGo Kids and Heal the Planet Together. I'm honored that Ken Fisher of Heal the Planet chose me as a Young Planet Leader, and I hope to do the title proud through my continued mental health education advocacy.

We have so many great experts on the Mindful Kids Peace Summit, and this book could not have happened without their quotes and teachings that I learned from our interviews, and I am grateful to them: Cory Alexander, guidance counselor, author, communication and social media; Lori Alhadeff, school board member, Keep Our Schools Safe, trauma; Laura Bakosh, Inner Explorer, mindfulness; Gina Biegel, Stressed Teens, MBSR-T; Knellee Bisram, AHAM Education, meditation; Karen Bluth, UNC professor, self-compassion; Michael Bready, Youth Mindfulness Kids, positive psychology; Chelsea Briggs, high school teacher at MSD Parkland; Debra Burdick, social worker, ADHD, The Brain Lady; Amy Burke, MindWell Education, education consultant, mindfulness; Richard Burnett, Mindfulness in Schools Project, professor; Patti Criswell, social worker, author; Sue DeCaro, parent coach, conscious living; Dan Devone, broadcaster, communication; Matt Dewar, high school teacher, 30,000 Pebbles; Amy Eva, Greater Good Science Center, kindness; Hazel Farrer, life coach; Dr. Jennifer Fraser, neuroscience and positive psychology; Dr. Diane Gehart, positive psychology, therapist; Sadiqa Glusman, nutritionist, Heal The Planet; Argos Gonzalez, high school teacher, Little Flower Yoga and Mindful Schools; Dr. Lee-Anne Gray, psychologist, trauma; Marnie Grundman, advocate, trafficking; Dr. Rick Hanson, psychologist and author, neuroscience and mindfulness; Dan Harris, broadcaster, meditation; Elayna Hasty, teen advocate, Girls Against Bullying; Kevin Hawkins, principal, MindWell Education, mindfulness; Dr. Sam Himmelstein, psychologist, Center for Adolescent Studies, trauma; Diamond Howard, Hanley Institute, substance abuse; Jon Kabat-Zinn, professor, author, Center for Mindfulness; Kid Capri, rapper, philanthropist; Heidi Kasevich, professor of leadership, Quiet Revolution; J.G. Larochette, middle school teacher, Mindful Life Project; Haris Lender, yoga, Kidding Around Yoga; Joe Lockett, radio show host and philanthropist; Helen Maffini, MindBE Education, mindfulness; Dr. Laura Martocci, psychologist, *Psychology Today*; Madison McEvoy, teen advocate, MSD Parkland; Ted Meissner, podcaster, Center for Mindfulness; Jennifer Miller, social-emotional learning, Confident Parents Confident Kids; Jenna Moniz, who was a guest on *The Better Mindset* podcast; Jessica Morey, Inward Bound Mindfulness Education, meditation; Andrew Jordan Nance, author, Mindful Arts San Francisco; Dr. Bradley Nelson, Discover Healing, the Emotion Code, releasing emotions; Orlaith O'Sullivan, the Calm Café, mindfulness; Alexandra Penn, Champions Against Bullying; Former US Congressman Tim Ryan, author, mindfulness; Dan Rechtschaffen, author, mindfulness; Sophie Riegel, teen advocate, mental health author; Maureik Robison, Inner Explorer, mindfulness; Ross Robinson, Holistic Life Foundation, meditation; Steve Ronik, Henderson Behavioral Health, substance abuse and suicide prevention; Bob Roth, David Lynch Foundation, meditation; Habib Sadeghi, holistic healing doctor, Be Hive for Healing and Love Buttons; Amy Saltzman, psychologist, Still Quiet Place; Sharon Salzberg, Insight Meditation Center, author; Heather Schwartz, Collaborative for Academic, Social Emotional Learning (CASEL); Supna Shah, WeGo Kids, Parent-TV, Emotional Intelligence; John Shearer, mindfulness coach; Nimrod Sheinman, naturopathic physician, Center for Mindfulness; Dr. Dan Siegel, psychiatrist, author, Mindsight

Institute; Emanuelle Sippy, teen advocate, self-awareness; Dave Smith, Mindful Schools, Secular Buddah, emotional intelligence; Heather Stang, thanatologist, mindfulness and grief; Whitney Stewart, mindful author; Jordan Temeres, teen advocate, MSD Parkland; Dave Trachtenberg, Walk the Middle Way, diversity and communication; Shelly Tygielsky, Pandemic of Love, Yuru meditation; Dr. Dzung Vo, pediatrician, *The Mindful Teen*; Dr. Regina Washington, formerly of LGBTQ Centerlink; Dr. Chris Willard, psychologist, Harvard Medical School professor, author, mindfulness; and Todd Wolfenberg, Yoga International.

I'm also grateful to Welbeck Publishing's Balance Imprint and Beth Bishop for taking a chance on me and believing that this book could ultimately help a teen or two somewhere out there. And for Soraya Nair and Andrea Marchiano of Trigger Publishing, who helped with the painstaking editing and all the you's vs. we's (inside joke). Thank you, too, to Gracie Kaplan-Stein and Shelly-Ann King, who are great connectors and awesome people. To Udonis Haslem, who is one of the coolest people I've ever met, thank you for believing in me and the message we are sending to teens in our community and all over the world.

Sometimes school and work collide, and there are people in my academic life who have been big supporters of my work, and I am thankful to each of them: former Broward County Superintendent Robert Runcie, who invited me to sit on the Superintendent's Mindfulness Initiative Committee; everyone in BCPS Student Support Services; my own amazing high school principal, Mrs. Perkovic; guidance counselors, Mrs. Dominguez, Mrs. Lily, Mr. Ziccardi and Mrs. Siwek; and teachers, who have guided me for four years, all of whom had my back, especially Mr. Berke, who was the sponsor of our mindfulness club, and Mr. Pichardo, my TV production advisor and mentor, who helped build my passion for journalism. I also want to thank my Posse family, our trainers, John and Anthony, and the rest of Posse 11, who are always in my corner.

There is a long list of family friends, school friends, work friends and personal friends, and I would like to thank every single one of them, but I think the publisher might get annoyed with the extra words, so I have to do a general thank-you to all of my incredible and awesome friends, many of whom I've known since preschool, and their families, who have treated me like their own, and who I know that I can always count on. You all know who you are. Thank you. All these people helped me with Wuf Shanti in some way and/or believed in me, listened to me and loved me. I hope to make a positive impact on the world and leave a legacy of advocacy, service and education.

All I know for sure is that change is constant. I am excited that I got accepted to Syracuse University as a Posse Scholar (where I may freeze, being Florida raised and moving to Upstate New York, where it can get to below zero degrees). Syracuse is one of the only universities with an undergraduate minor in mindfulness, so being at this school will allow me to continue to work on my two passions of sports journalism and mental health. I'm not sure what the future holds or if I'll want to do this forever, but I know whatever I do, it'll be something I love and something that helps others. For everyone who has helped me become who I am today and who will support me in whatever future endeavors I choose, I thank you, and I'm grateful.

RESOURCES

The resources here are not an exhaustive list, but these are just some of the many wonderful organizations that can support you.

> **If you need help, don't hesitate to reach out.**

US MENTAL HEALTH CRISIS RESOURCES:
- 988 Suicide & Crisis Lifeline: **Call or text 988**
  - *Ayuda en español*: **1-888-628-9454**
  - Veterans Crisis Line: **Call 988 or text 838255**
  - For the deaf and hard of hearing: **Use your preferred relay service or dial 711, then 988**
- National Crisis Text Line: **Text HOME to 741741**
- The Trevor Project (LGBTQ+): **Call 1-866-488-7386 or text START to 678678**
- National Domestic Violence Hotline: **1-800-799-7233**
- Women in Distress 24-Hour Crisis Hotline (for anyone experiencing domestic violence): **954-761-1133**
- Substance Abuse and Mental Health Services Administration (SAMHSA) Helpline: **1-800-662-4357**
- National Eating Disorder Association Helpline: **Call or text 1-800-931-2237**
- National Alliance on Mental Illness (NAMI) Helpline (for cutting/self-harm): **Call or text 1-800-950-6264**
- National Runaway Hotline: **1-800-RUNAWAY (1-800-786-2929)**

INTERNATIONAL MENTAL HEALTH CRISIS RESOURCES:

- UK and Ireland: **Call 116 123 or text SHOUT to 85258**
- Canada: **Call 1-833-456-4566 or text 45645**
- Australia: **Call 13 11 14**
- If your country isn't listed above, check this list of international hotlines: **https://blog.opencounseling.com/suicide-hotlines/**

OTHER MENTAL HEALTH AND WELL-BEING RESOURCES:

- World Health Organization: **https://www.who.int**
- National Alliance on Mental Illness (NAMI): **https://www.nami.org**
- American Psychiatric Association: **https://www.psychiatry.org/**

MINDFULNESS RESOURCES:

- Wuf Shanti Children's Wellness Foundation/Mindful Kids Peace Summit: **https://wufshanti.com**
- Wuf Shanti's YouTube Channel: **https://www.youtube.com/c/WufShanti/videos**
- Inner Explorer: **https://innerexplorer.org/**
- Heal The Planet: **https://healtheplanet.com**
- Stressed Teens: **https://stressedteens.com**
- Public Service Announcements for Teens: **https://wufshanti.com/mindful-kids-peace- summit-psas/**
- Kids Association for Mindfulness in Education, which brings youth together to mindfully do good in the world and help get mindful programs into schools: **http://www.mindfuleducation.org/kame/**
- *Mindful* magazine: **https://www.mindful.org/peace-begins-with-me/**

SOCIAL-EMOTIONAL LEARNING (SEL) RESOURCES:

- Collaborative for Academic, Social, Emotional Learning (CASEL): **https://casel.org/**
- MindBE Education: MBSEL trainings, curriculum, and programs **https://mindbe-education.com/**
- Greater Good at UC Berkeley: Science based insights for a meaningful life **https://greatergood.berkeley.edu/**

FOR MORE INFORMATION ABOUT THE UDONIS HASLEM FOUNDATION:
https://www.udcares.org/

MY TEDX TALK ON MINDFULNESS:
https://www.ted.com/talks/adam_avin_mindfulness_in_ education_to_lower_stress_and_violence

MY KEYNOTE SPEECH AT THE BROWARD MENTAL HEALTH SUMMIT:
https://www.youtube.com/watch?v=xFbe6hgalbc

INDEX OF ACTIVITIES

REFERENCES

1   Zraick, K. (2019, February 20). *Teenagers Say Depression and Anxiety Are Major Issues Among Their Peers*. The New York Times. Retrieved December 2020, from https://www.nytimes.com/2019/02/20/health/teenage-depression-statistics.html

2   Avin, A. (2019). *Adam Avin: Mindfulness in Education to Lower Stress and Violence | TED Talk*. Retrieved December 2020, from https://www.ted.com/talks/adam_avin_mindfulness_in_education_to_lower_stress_and_violence

3   Common Sense Media. (2021, March). *The Common Sense Census: Media Use by Teens and Tweens*. Retrieved from https://www.commonsensemedia.org/sites/default/files/research/report/8-18-census-integrated-report-final-web_0.pdf

4   *What is the Casel Framework?* CASEL. (n.d.). Retrieved December 2020, from https://casel.org/sel-framework/

5   *What is the Casel Framework?* CASEL. (n.d.). Retrieved December 2020, from https://casel.org/sel-framework/

6   *What is the Casel Framework?* CASEL. (n.d.). Retrieved December 2020, from https://casel.org/sel-framework/

7   *What is the Casel Framework?* CASEL. (n.d.). Retrieved December 2020, from https://casel.org/sel-framework/

8   *What is the Casel Framework?* CASEL. (n.d.). Retrieved December 2020, from https://casel.org/sel-framework/

9   Goodreads. (n.d.). *A Quote by Maya Angelou*. Goodreads. Retrieved January 2023, from https://www.goodreads.com/quotes/7532767-forgive-yourself-for-not-knowing-what-you-didn-t-know-before

10 Stoner, K. (2019, October 1). *Science Proves That What Doesn't Kill You Makes You Stronger*. Northwestern Now. Retrieved December 2020, from https://news.northwestern.edu/stories/2019/10/science-proves-that-what-doesnt-kill-you-makes-you-stronger/

11 Bastian, B. (2019, February 20). *The Resilience Paradox: Why We Often Get Resilience Wrong*. Psychology Today. Retrieved November 2020, from https://www.psychologytoday.com/us/blog/the-other-side/201902/the-resilience-paradox-why-we-often-get-resilience-wrong

12 American Psychological Association. (n.d.). *Resilience*. Retrieved November 2020, from https://www.apa.org/topics/resilience/

13 STOMP Out Bullying. (n.d.). *The Issue of Bullying*. Retrieved December 2020, from https://www.stompoutbullying.org/issue-bullying

14 Zraick, K. (2019, February 20). *Teenagers Say Depression and Anxiety Are Major Issues Among Their Peers*. The New York Times. Retrieved December 2020, from https://www.nytimes.com/2019/02/20/health/teenage-depression-statistics.html

15 Centers for Disease Control and Prevention. (2022, June 3). *Data and Statistics on Children's Mental Health.* Retrieved 2022, from https://www.cdc.gov/childrensmentalhealth/data.html

16 Merriam-Webster. (n.d.). Depression. Retrieved November 2020, from https://www.merriam-webster.com/dictionary/depression

17 Taylor, J. (2016, December 26). *20 Wayne Dyer Quotes About Life.* Jane Taylor I Mindfulness & Compassion Teacher I Mind-Body Connection Coach I Wellbeing Coaching I Mindful Self-Compassion Coaching I Gold Coast. Retrieved November 2020, from https://www.habitsforwellbeing.com/20-wayne-dyer-quotes-about-life/

18 *Learn.* Jack.org. (n.d.). Retrieved 2020, from https://jack.org/Resources/Learn

19 Underwood, N. (2020, April 14). *The Teenage Brain.* Retrieved 2020 from https://thewalrus.ca/the-teenage-brain/

20 BBC. (2019, March 19). *People Don't Become 'Adults' Until Their 30s, Say Scientists.* BBC News. Retrieved January 2023, from https://www.bbc.co.uk/news/newsbeat-47622059

21 Nardino, M. (2022, March 29). *Simone Biles' Most Honest Quotes About Mental Health and Wellness.* Us Weekly. Retrieved 2022, from https://www.usmagazine.com/celebrity-news/pictures/simone-biles-most-honest-quotes-about-mental-health-wellness/

22 Boyle, J. (2022, May 31). *Seahawks Launch Mental Health Matters Program.* Seahawks.com. Retrieved 2022, from https://www.seahawks.com/news/seahawks-launch-mental-health-matters-program

23 Buford, L. (2020, May 2). *How Mental Conditioning Has Guided Seahawks QB Russell Wilson to Sustained Success.* Retrieved 2022, from https://www.si.com/nfl/seahawks/news/how-mental-conditioning-has-guided-seahawks-qb-russell-wilson-to-sustained-success

24 Calm. (2019, December 11). Facebook. Retrieved 2022, from https://www.facebook.com/calm/photos/a.599922303392257/2928156003902197/?type=3&locale2=ja_JP&paipv=0&eav=AfaUbTTL9iRPwEc6fezbxNah0Inl8_JZLh_YtnxU5BOEADNHJmqGgtB65vLZlMdSq6Y&_rdr

25 Adler, M. (2015, April 11). *Spieth's Instructor Since Age 12 Knew He Had Something Special.* The Loop. Retrieved 2022, from https://www.golfdigest.com/story/spieths-instructor-since-age-1

26 *About Us.* Kevin Love Fund. (n.d.). Retrieved 2022, from https://kevinlovefund.org/about-us/

27 Love, K. (2022, February 28). *Everyone is Going Through Something.* The Players' Tribune. Retrieved 2022, from https://www.theplayerstribune.com/articles/kevin-love-everyone-is-going-through-something

28 *Our Approach.* Jack.org. (n.d.). Retrieved January 2023, from https://jack.org/About/Our-Approach

29 AACAP. (2011, December). Understanding Violent Behavior in Children and Adolescents. Retrieved November 2020, from https://www.aacap.org/AACAP/Families_and_Youth/Facts_for_Families/FFF-Guide/Understanding-Violent-Behavior-In-Children-and-Adolescents-55.aspx

REFERENCES

30 Dr. Irminne Van Dyken. (2019). *Nasal Nitric Oxide: Can you HUM your way to better health?* Retrieved 2020, from https://www.youtube.com/watch?v=6v-nTRLEXFk.

31 Team, B. and S. (2023, January 6). *How to Turn Around Your Negative Thinking.* Cleveland Clinic. Retrieved January 2023, from https://health.clevelandclinic.org/turn-around-negative-thinking/

32 What is a Mandala? (n.d.). Retrieved November 2020, from http://www.mandalaproject.org/What/Index.html

33 *Meditation Quote 63.* Daily Meditate. (2014, June 24). Retrieved November 2020, from https://dailymeditate.com/meditation-quote-63-if-every-8-year-old-in-the-world-is-taught-meditation-we-will-eliminate-violence-from-the-world-within-one-generation-dalai-lama/

34 Kabat-Zinn, J. (2019). *Broward County Workshop.*

35 Heffernan, A., & Lillegraven, T. (2013, January 24). *Adam Levine's Yoga Workout.* Retrieved November 2020, from https://www.menshealth.com/fitness/g19537449/adam-levine-stretches/

36 Griffin, J. H. (1996). *Black Like Me.* Signet.

37 US Department of Health and Human Services. (n.d.). *I'm So Stressed Out! Fact Sheet.* National Institute of Mental Health. Retrieved December 2020, from https://www.nimh.nih.gov/health/publications/stress/index.shtml

38 Burdick, D. (2018). *Wuf Shanti Mindful Kids Peace Summit.*

39 Willard, C. (n.d.). Facebook. Retrieved November 2020, from https://www.facebook.com/drchriswillard

40 *About Us.* Inner Explorer. (n.d.). Retrieved January 2023, from https://innerexplorer.org/aboutus

This book also contains quotes from the following interviews conducted by me, Helen Maffini or both of us at the Wuf Shanti Mindful Kids Peace Summit:

Alexandra Penn (2018)

Amy Burke (2019)

Amy Eva (2018)

Dr. Amy Saltzman (2018)

Andrew Jordan Nance (2019)

Argos Gonzalez (2018, 2019)

Bob Roth (2018, 2019)

Dr. Bradley Nelson (2020)

Chelsea Briggs (2019)

Dr. Chris Willard (2018)

Cory Alexander (2018, 2019)

Dan Devone (2019, 2020)

Dan Harris (2019, 2020)

Dr. Dan Siegel (2019)

Dave Smith (2018, 2019)

Dave Trachtenberg (2018, 2019)

Diamond Howard (2019)

Dr. Diane Gehart (2018, 2019)

Dr. Dzung Vo (2018, 2019)

Elayna Hasty (2019)

Emanuelle Sippy (2019)

Emily Brierly (2019)

Gina Biegel (2019)

Haris Lender (2017)

Heather Schwartz (2018, 2019)

Heather Stang (2018)

Helen Maffini (2020)

J.G. Larochette (2020)

Jenna Moniz (2021)

Jennifer Miller (2018, 2019)

Jessica Morey (2019)

Joe Lockett (2017, 2018)

Jordan Temeres (2018, 2019)

Karen Bluth (2018)

Kevin Hawkins (2019)

Laura Bakosh (2019, 2020)

Dr. Laura Martocci (2019)

Laurie Rich-Levinson (2019)

Dr. Lee-Anne Gray (2019)

Lori Alhadeff (2019)

Madison McEvoy (2018, 2019)

Marnie Grundman (2020)

Matt Dewar (2018, 2019)

Maureik Robison (2018, 2019)

Orlaith O'Sullivan (2018)

REFERENCES

Patti Criswell (2018)

Dr. Regina Washington (2019, 2020)

Dr. Rick Hanson (2019)

Robert Runcie (2019)

Ross Robinson (2018, 2019)

Sadiqa Glusman (2019)

Dr. Sam Himmelstein (2018, 2019)

Shelly Tygielsky (2019, 2020)

Sophie Riegel (2019)

Steve Ronik (2019, 2020)

Sue DeCaro (2019)

Supna Shah (2017, 2018)

Tim Ryan (2017, 2019)

Todd Wolfenberg (2019)

Whitney Stewart (2018)

You can find the Wuf Shanti Mindful Peace Summit interviews via YouTube.

TriggerHub.org is one of the most elite and scientifically proven forms of mental health intervention

Trigger Publishing is the leading independent mental health and wellbeing publisher in the UK and US. Our collection of bibliotherapeutic books and the power of lived experience change lives forever. Our courageous authors' lived experiences and the power of their stories are scientifically endorsed by independent federal, state and privately funded research in the US. These stories are intrinsic elements in reducing stigma, making those with poor mental health feel less alone, giving them the privacy they need to heal, ensuring they are guided by the essential steps to kick-start their own journeys to recovery, and providing hope and inspiration when they need it most.

Clinical and scientific research conducted by assistant professor Dr Kristin Kosyluk and her highly acclaimed team in the Department of Mental Health Law & Policy at the University of South Florida (USF), as well as complementary research by her peers across the US, has independently verified the power of lived experience as a core component in achieving mental health prosperity. Their findings categorically confirm lived experience as a leading method in treating those struggling with poor mental health by significantly reducing stigma and the time it takes for them to seek help, self-help or signposting if they are struggling.

Delivered through TriggerHub, our unique online portal and smartphone app, we make our library of bibliotherapeutic titles and other vital resources accessible to individuals and organizations anywhere, at any time and with complete privacy, a crucial element of recovery. As such, TriggerHub is the primary recommendation across the UK and US for the delivery of lived experiences.

At Trigger Publishing and TriggerHub, we proudly lead the way in making the unseen become seen. We are dedicated to humanizing mental health, breaking stigma and challenging outdated societal values to create real action and impact. Find out more about our world-leading work with lived experience and bibliotherapy via triggerhub.org, or by joining us on:

- 🐦 @triggerhub_
- ⓕ @triggerhub.org
- 📷 @triggerhub_

Dr Kristin Kosyluk, Ph.D., is an assistant professor in the Department of Mental Health Law and Policy at USF, a faculty affiliate of the Louis de la Parte Florida Mental Health Institute, and director of the STigma Action Research (STAR) Lab. Find out more about Dr Kristin Kosyluk, her team and their work by visiting:

USF Department of Mental Health Law & Policy:
www.usf.edu/cbcs/mhlp/index.aspx

USF College of Behavioral and Community Sciences:
www.usf.edu/cbcs/index.aspx

STAR Lab: www.usf.edu/cbcs/mhlp/centers/star-lab/

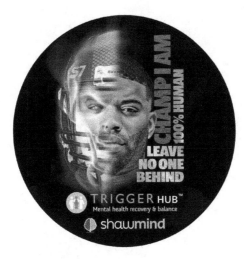

Printed in the USA
CPSIA information can be obtained
at www.ICGtesting.com
JSHW011344180624
65043JS00004B/200